CONTENTS

Olivia Arezzolo is a leading sleep expert in Australia. After nine years of study, Olivia's qualifications include a Bachelor of Social Science (Psychology), Certificate of Sleep Psychology, Diploma of Health Science (Nutritional Medicine) and a Certificate 3+4 in Fitness. She has been featured in *Forbes Magazines* and on BBC Radio and *The Today Show*, and partnered with global brands such as Tempur-Pedic and Ikea. Her core mission is to improve the lives of everyone – inside and out – and she is doing so via the vehicle of sleep. She lives in Bondi Beach, Australia. You can connect with Olivia via her website, oliviaarezzolo.com.au.

BEAR,
LION
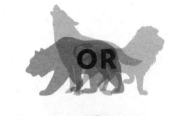
OR
WOLF

**How Understanding Your Sleep-type
Could Change Your Life**

OLIVIA AREZZOLO

First published in the UK by Lagom
An imprint of Bonnier Books UK
4th Floor, Victoria House,
Bloomsbury Square,
London, WC1B 4DA

Owned by Bonnier Books
Sveavägen 56, Stockholm, Sweden

Paperback: 978-1-7887-0453-3
Ebook: 978-1-7887-0454-0

A CIP catalogue of this book is available from the British Library.

Designed and typeset by Envy Design
Printed and bound by Clays Ltd, Elcograf S.p.A

1 3 5 7 9 10 8 6 4 2

Lagom is an imprint of Bonnier Books UK
www.bonnierbooks.co.uk

INTRODUCTION

You may wonder, did I suffer from insomnia – is that why I got into sleep? Or did I just have a passion for it? To be honest, I didn't suffer from insomnia, but I have suffered extremely poor mental and physical health – which led me to where I am today, and to writing this book.

At the tender age of fourteen, I suffered from major depression, including a suicide attempt. Years of ongoing struggle had evolved into bulimia by the age of fifteen, and then anorexia at sixteen – the latter granting me a six-week hospital stint and three months of outpatient treatment. Although being in hospital was a low point, it was also my *turning* point.

One night in hospital, at the age of seventeen, I wanted to go to a friend's birthday party but the team responsible for my care wouldn't let me out. It was awful. Then it dawned on me: *If I don't get better, I will miss out on life.* I can still remember that moment very clearly: it was the moment I decided to commit to recovery and choose life over death, light over dark.

And with that decision, everything changed. Food? I ate it. Therapists? I went to all the appointments. Negative thoughts? I beat them down with a ten-foot pole. A few months later, I was steaming ahead with my recovery. When I do something, I do it *properly*. And, in the process, I got my life back: memories, joy, laughter, friendship, connection to community and more. I very quickly went from my darkest dark to my best self – and loved feeling happy, healthy and content once more.

If you're wondering what this has to do with helping people sleep, stay with me. Essentially, by getting my life back after being so sick, I knew my purpose was to help others do the same. So, when I finished school, I studied a range of degrees in the wellness space – psychology, nutrition, sleep and fitness – and started coaching.

Initially, I helped clients with a range of concerns – stress, weight loss, motivation – and then sleep. Thanks to my advice, my sleep clients saw rapid, transformative results – so, more and more, I became a 'go-to' sleep guru.

After a few months, I knew I was onto something – not only were new sleep clients coming at me left, right and centre, I was approached by global brands Sealy Posturepedic and Ikea to be their media spokesperson. I tell you, if there was ever any doubt in my mind that I'd found my 'thing', it disappeared when two of the biggest companies in the bedding world popped into my inbox, completely out of the blue, and asked me to represent them.

That was 2018. Since then, I've been featured in *Forbes* magazine – a career highlight, definitely – appeared multiple times on *The Today Show* and been interviewed on BBC Radio.

Media aside, I've helped my clients and the wider community sleep better, and ultimately, reclaim their lives – exactly as I set out to at the age of seventeen.

As I worked with my clients, I noticed many of them had distinct preferences to go to sleep and wake at particular times. After researching the area, I realised this was the concept of a *chronotype* (a classification system – Bear, Wolf or Lion – that's used to help understand sleep and productivity cycles). I discovered that when I adapted my strategies to my client's specific sleep chronotype, they enjoyed even greater results – in particular, they were able to fall asleep faster, sleep deeper and wake up more refreshed.

Before we go any further, here's a very quick overview of the chronotypes. Lions like to go to sleep and wake the earliest. They tend to be 'A types' and natural-born leaders who are positive, proactive and goal-oriented. Bears like to rise later than Lions (and often hit an energy slump at around 3pm), but are known for being level-headed, generous, humble and reliable. Wolves like to go to bed and rise latest of all – they are the night owls of the chronotype world. They can be fun-loving and sociable but are also prone to anxiety and stress.

If you've come across chronotypes before, you may have heard of a fourth: the Dolphin. This chronotype has been used to categorise people who suffer from fatigue, have extreme personality tendencies and often face myriad health challenges posed by insufficient sleep (such as anxiety disorders, depression, weight problems and diabetes). However, I have chosen to intentionally leave out the Dolphin chronotype from this book. Based on my own research and experiences with my clients, I believe the Dolphin is actually more likely to be an extreme version of the Wolf.

The success I enjoyed using chronotypes with my sleep clients inspired me to organise *my* schedule according to my chronotype too – and before you ask, I'm a Lion who likes to go to sleep and rise early. As our chronotype predicts when we are most productive, I also shifted my work hours – and was able to get more done in less time. In addition, it helped me map out when to exercise, eat, socialise and even have sex – and again, I saw great results. Consequently, I now show up as my best self in every situation, work and personal life included.

Identifying and understanding chronotypes has also been an asset for my relationships. My mum, who is a Bear, isn't as fresh as I am in the morning, so when visiting I know to give her a little extra space and make her a coffee after we've finished our meditation. Similarly, for my Wolf friends, I don't hold it against them if they dip out from our 6am walk – I know it doesn't align with their circadian rhythm.

With the above in mind, I believe we *all* need to know our chronotype, as it helps us sleep better, feel better, and ultimately, *live* better. If that's what you're eager to do, know that you're in the right place. All I ask is that you trust the process, follow the plan and reach out for support if you need – I'm only an email away (check out my website, oliviaarezzolo.com.au). But please note, although I'm passionate about helping people with sleep, I am not a medical professional, so it's best to always seek the advice of your doctor and/or specialist before embarking on any course of supplements or making any significant dietary or lifestyle changes.

Before you go any further, please grab a highlighter and notepad. As you are reading through the book, jot down key insights or takeaways, points of relevance and any thoughts you'd like to pass on to your nearest and dearest. Given that sleep deprivation now affects around eight out of ten of us, most of the people you care about probably want to sleep better too. In fact, I encourage you to apply these teachings to your own life first, and when you see the results, which I know you will, share them with others. The thing is, you won't even have to try. By becoming the best version of yourself, you'll inspire others to do the same.

Not only is this a beautiful gift to impart to those around you, you'll also be helping me in my own personal mission: to help others feel their best inside and out via the vehicle of sleep. Together, I have no doubt, we can be unstoppable.

Enjoy the read, and sleep well.

PART 1

HOW WELL DO YOU SLEEP?

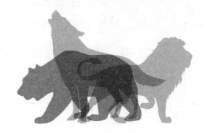

1

THE SCIENCE OF SLEEP

Sleep – our favourite pastime. Waking from a deep, rejuvenating rest, feeling mentally fresh, fired up and ready to go – remember that? Or those times you open your eyes and realise you have slept through the whole night, barely moved an inch, and feel like you could take on the world – feels good, doesn't it?

Unfortunately, as a sleep coach, I know for many of us, this just isn't happening. Instead, our experience with sleep is . . . well . . . not so enlivening, to say the least. Marred with bedtime anxiety, nighttime wakings and feeling less refreshed than when you went to sleep, for many of us, sleep is just not what it used to be.

If that's resonating with you, then first, I'm sorry for your experience. After years of working with clients who are facing problems sleeping, I fully appreciate how debilitating this can be: from feeling constantly on edge and unable to mentally switch off, through having such bad brain fog that you can't even remember where you put your keys, to that constant, undulating exhaustion accompanying only a few hours of proper rest. I am all too aware that sleeplessness isn't just a problem at night. Rather, it is a problem that affects every aspect of your life.

At the same time, I'm so pleased you're here. You are in exactly the right place you need to be and I am the coach you need to see lasting, real and radical change.

Even if it feels like you've tried everything, that all hope is lost and nothing will *actually* work, I'm here to let you know you haven't tried this yet. That is, my science-based strategy to improve sleep, based on your biology – your chronotype. Second to that, you haven't had my structure to show you how to make your new habits stick – a challenge for us all, myself included. Nor have you had my support.

So, in fact, you haven't tried *everything*. So it's entirely possible that this solution is the one for you. This has been the case time and time again for my clients, who come to me with exactly the same hesitation and thought patterns as you may well be experiencing right now and, literally, within a matter of weeks, they are sleeping properly again.

Clients like Dave,* who was a DJ in his younger years and was unable to sleep longer than four hours. Within weeks, he was sleeping seven hours. Or Sally,* whose bedtime anxiety became so bad that the only way she could fall asleep was to use sleeping pills. After two sessions, she was able to fall asleep within fifteen minutes. Or perhaps Jessie,* who was waking four times every night, struggling to return to sleep. Within two weeks of us working together, she was waking only once to use the bathroom and able to fall back to sleep straight away.

Each of these clients thought that nothing would ever change and they were destined for a life of mental fogginess and fatigue. Then, they trusted in my guidance, followed the plan and, within weeks, were able to sleep somewhat normally again. It happened to them and it can happen to you. All you need to do is trust the process, follow the plan and reach out for support should things get tough (because at some point, they probably will).

---

* Note: names of clients have been changed to protect their privacy

I'm here for you in the good times, the bad times and the rollercoaster that's often somewhere in between.

First up, we need to know a little more about sleep science. This will build the foundation you need to see the change you so desperately want: sleeping longer, sleeping deeper and waking up more refreshed.

So, without further ado, let's get started.

SLEEP DEPRIVATION

Some of us know only too well that we are sleep deprived. Signs like constant exhaustion, a reliance on caffeine and feeling 'wired but tired' are part of our daily experience. However, others may not be so aware. I mean, who's to say it's not normal to feel fatigued most mornings? Do we feel stressed and anxious because we live in a 24/7 society or is it a sign of sub-par sleep? Is being unproductive something to do with sleep quality or perhaps just a matter of lack of interest in your work?

To start, I'm going to share the common signs of sleep deprivation so you can know, without any uncertainty, if your sleep needs to be addressed. Before I do, though, please note that just because it's widespread, it doesn't mean it isn't a problem. After all, research shows that

77 per cent of us sleep insufficiently on a weekly basis. That means most of us are actually sleep deprived and will be experiencing some, if not all, of these symptoms.

1. Feeling constantly fatigued

If there is one indication that you haven't slept enough, it's feeling so tired that walking to the kitchen to make a cup of coffee seems hard. If you're working full time, this is likely to be you. Seven in ten full-time workers attain less than six hours of sleep each night and 40 per cent report severe daytime fatigue on a weekly basis. Wolves – research shows you have the least sleep, so if anyone's going to be foggy and fatigued, it's you. However, Bears aren't too far behind you. Lions – you sleep the most, so are least likely to suffer from fatigue.

2. Making more mistakes than usual

Put salt instead of sugar in your coffee this morning? Or perhaps you tried to start the car with your house keys? Or maybe you took the wrong lunch to work without realising it? I've heard these tales time and time again from my sleep-deprived clients. If this is resonating with you, take the weight off your shoulders and know that, when sleep deprived, such mistakes are completely normal.

Lack of sleep impairs your frontal lobe – the brain region responsible for decision making, judgement and time management. A 2016 sleep survey by Australia's Sleep Health Foundation found that 29 per cent of workplace errors can be directly attributed to fatigue – yes, that's almost one in three. If that's you, please do not feel like there is something wrong with you. Your body is just trying to communicate to you, '*I need more sleep*'.

3. Brain fog and memory loss

Alongside more mistakes, memory loss is a natural consequence of inadequate sleep. For each night you don't sleep enough, your levels of beta-amyloid (Aβ), a neurotoxin that contributes to brain fog, impaired memory and even Alzheimer's disease, increases by 5 per cent. Yes, you read that correctly. This happens *each night*, let alone after weeks, months or years of insufficient sleep.

4. Being unproductive

Being productive is something we all want, but when we're sleep deprived, boy, is it tough to achieve. According to a 2017 study published in the *American Journal of Health Promotion*, sleeping less than five hours makes us four times less productive. That means a ten-minute task can take forty! This really puts things into perspective around staying up late to get ahead on tomorrow's work, doesn't it? This would be particularly irritating to hard-working Bears, who typically have a 'can-do' attitude. Unfortunately, when sleep deprived, saying 'yes' to every task thrown at you becomes near impossible – as I am sure many of us would understand.

5. Feeling anxious and being unable to 'switch off'

Anxiety is a massive problem in our society. According to the mental health organisation Beyond Blue, one in four people will experience anxiety at some stage in their life – it's something I personally face too. And, yes, sleep loss is a major contributing factor. Research by the University of Chicago found that just *one* night of insufficient sleep can see the stress hormone cortisol increase by 37 per cent. After two nights, it's 45 per cent. The consequences of this include an inability to switch off, feeling 'wired but tired' and mental rumination. The problem is, as you probably know, this perpetuates a cycle of sleeplessness – insufficient sleep increases anxiety, making it harder to fall and stay asleep, which then increases anxiety even further. In terms of chronotypes, according to a 2020 study featured in the peer-reviewed journal *PLOS One*,

Wolves are statistically the most likely to be anxious, but that doesn't mean that Lions and Bears don't suffer from anxiety too.

6. Impaired immunity

In light of the Covid-19 pandemic, we should all be looking to boost our immune system to protect ourselves and the ones we love. However, when sleep deprived, this isn't so easy. In fact, research led by the University of California in 2015 found that you are over four times more likely to catch a cold when you're sleeping six rather than seven hours at night. Yes, just one hour less of sleep escalates your risk of becoming unwell by around four times.

7. Weight gain and sugar cravings

Ah, that mid-morning muffin! Or that 3pm visit to your corner store to see what chocolate bar takes your fancy. Or a bit of both. Right? Trust me, it's not *just* you. These sugar cravings are extremely normal, almost to be expected, when we are sleep deprived. A 2004 study led by the University of Chicago found that sugar cravings increase by as much as 45 per cent after only two nights of insufficient sleep. In addition, you also have a 28 per cent increase in the hunger hormone ghrelin and an

18 per cent decrease in the satiety hormone leptin. This means you're hungrier, less satisfied when you do eat and specifically craving sugar. So next time you struggle to keep your hands out of the cookie jar at work and feel guilty, don't – you might just be sleep deprived.

As you can see, there is more to sleep deprivation than just being fatigued. It's the brain fog, the memory lapses, the anxiety and the lack of productivity. Essentially, it's the loss of you being you. You become a different version of yourself. One who is tired, wired, fed up and, all in all, just wanting to get some sleep. Trust me, I can fully appreciate this.

Though I haven't had sleep issues, I have had anxiety issues and I understand how frustrating, debilitating and limiting it can be. You are literally unable to live your life. I'm also aware that when I was really unwell, I would have given *anything* to take away those feelings. I'm sure this will resonate with many of you.

THE ARCHITECTURE OF SLEEP

At this point, I'm sure you're asking, *Why can I sleep for eight hours but still feel exhausted?* This all comes down to sleep quality. Just because you are sleeping, it doesn't mean you are sleeping *well*. Quantity does not equate to quality.

Essentially, not all sleep is the same: there's light sleep (stage 1 NREM), which is when we are almost semi-conscious; slightly deeper sleep (stage 2 NREM), when you're slightly harder to wake; then deep sleep (stage 3+4 NREM, also known as slow-wave sleep or SWS). Deep sleep is where the gold is – it's what helps us feel truly rejuvenated upon waking.

That's a brief overview of the different parts of sleep. Now let's explore a little more about each stage ...

Stage 1 NREM

Ideally, you want to spend only 5 per cent of your total sleep time here. In this stage, we are easily woken and it's not overly refreshing. If you are easily disturbed by noise or sound, you're probably in this sleep stage. Brainwaves seen in this stage are primarily alpha.

Stage 2 NREM

This sleep stage is slightly deeper than stage 1 and it (optimally) accounts for 50 per cent of your total sleep time. In this stage, we're harder to wake than stage 1 and see slower brainwaves.

Occurring in this sleep stage are phenomena called sleep spindles, which are important for learning and memory. Sleep spindles indicate we are encoding new information into long-term memory. A 2002 study in the *Journal of Neuroscience* found that after a day of learning, sleep spindle activity was 34 per cent higher than usual that night.

Stage 3+4 NREM (SWS)

Stage 3+4 NREM or slow-wave sleep (SWS) is the all-important deep sleep stage. It is marked by super slow, delta brainwaves and if you are lucky, you will spend 20 per cent of your total sleep time here. SWS usually occurs in the first two-thirds of the night (typically before 3am) and is critical for both mental and physical recovery.

In terms of physical recovery, it's during SWS that 70 per cent of human growth hormone (HGH) is produced, the primary hormone responsible for cellular repair and recovery. If you've slept for eight hours and have woken exhausted, there's a good chance your body hasn't produced enough HGH, nor have you spent enough time in SWS.

In terms of mental recovery, SWS is equally important as this is when beta-amyloid (Aβ) detoxification takes place. As I mentioned earlier, Aβ is a neurotoxin and the process of eliminating it improves mental clarity and memory retention. If our body doesn't eliminate enough Aβ, it could increase our risk of Alzheimer's disease – Aβ plaques in the brain are a hallmark sign of the illness.

Another feature of SWS is sleep inertia – waking up groggy, almost as if you were drunk. If you're awakened during this stage, you may feel extremely disoriented, foggy and fatigued. This is exactly why you don't want to nap for longer than 30 minutes – if you do, you may enter SWS and end up feeling worse than you did before the nap.

With respect to chronotypes, Wolves should take note – your natural preference for a late bedtime means you run the risk of inadequate SWS.

REM sleep

The last stage of sleep we will discuss is REM sleep. While both SWS and REM sleep are deep-sleep stages, they are, in fact, very different. Unlike SWS, during REM sleep the body produces highly active brainwaves, such as alpha, beta and gamma. Also unlike SWS, REM sleep occurs in the last third of the night (typically after 3am). We should aim to spend 25 per cent of our sleeping time here.

Three things in particular are happening during REM sleep: memory consolidation, dreams and emotional regulation.

Let's look at memory consolidation first. While both SWS and REM sleep are important to memory, this is for different reasons. During SWS, we encode declarative, location and visual memories (for example, knowing the name of something and where it is); during REM sleep, we encode procedural memories (knowing *how* to do something).

Next, dreams. Scientists have established that we dream while in REM sleep, but there's still a lack of clarity as to *why* we do it. (So if you were about to ask about the purpose of dreams, I'm sorry, I don't have an answer for you! However, it is possible that dreams are linked to emotional regulation as both occur during REM sleep.)

Finally, emotional regulation. Essentially, we need REM sleep for emotional stability. A 2012 clinical trial published in *Frontiers of Neuroscience* found that depriving individuals of REM sleep (allowing them to experience only 4 per cent of their total sleep time in REM sleep rather than an adequate 21 per cent) made them more emotionally reactive. And while it's reasonable to think this was perhaps due to total sleep loss, it wasn't. The study also included a group of participants deprived of the other sleep stages who weren't as emotionally reactive. The results indicated that it was lack of REM sleep specifically that led to emotional instability.

The chronotype most at risk for inadequate REM is Wolves, as they typically sleep for the least amount of time. The body prioritises SWS first, so if you're not sleeping for long enough, you're unlikely to attain adequate REM sleep.

OPTIMAL TIME PROPORTION FOR EACH SLEEP STAGE

5 per cent: stage 1 NREM

50 per cent: stage 2 NREM

20 per cent: stage 3+4 NREM, SWS

25 per cent: REM

Now that you have an understanding of sleep stages, let's move ahead to something a little more juicy: the ins and outs of your chronotype. To start, we'll learn about the circadian rhythm, which as you'll see, is inherently intertwined with your sleep personality.

CIRCADIAN RHYTHM – DANCING TO THE TUNE OF YOUR OWN BODY

'Circadian rhythm' is a term that is often passed around but, if you are like I was before I specialised in sleep, you may not really understand it, so let me explain what it is. In the simplest terms, the circadian rhythm is our twenty-four-hour body clock responsible for our sleep–wake cycle. It's primarily controlled by two factors: our daily external twenty-four-hour clock (as in the light–dark cycle) and our own internal twenty-four-hour clock. Ideally, these two clocks match and, as a result, our bodies produce melatonin (the sleep hormone) during the evening and suppress this hormone during the day.

However, the two clocks don't always match – and this results in circadian misalignment and sleeping difficulties. As many Wolves would know, although the external clock may signal it is time for sleep (that is, it is dark outside), our internal clock may signal it's not time to produce melatonin yet and subsequently we feel wide awake. This is exactly why many Wolves find it hard to fall asleep – they have a circadian misalignment.

> ## THE LOWDOWN ON MELATONIN
>
> The 'master' sleep hormone, melatonin helps us fall and stay asleep. Its production is controlled by the circadian rhythm and, therefore, primarily by light. In the absence of light, melatonin is produced and we feel sleepy; in the presence of light, melatonin is suppressed and we feel alert. As the circadian rhythm operates on a twenty-four-hour cycle, so too does melatonin, which is why each night we feel tired at roughly the same time, and in the morning, we feel alert at roughly around the same time.
>
> Melatonin can be taken in pill form as a sleep supplement – we'll discuss this more in chapter eight.

YOUR CHRONOTYPE

Understanding your chronotype is pivotal to you sleeping properly. Not doing so could be the reason why nothing has worked until now. In the simplest of terms, chronotypes are the biological disposition to rise and sleep at certain times and are indicative of your underlying circadian preferences. As discussed, I categorised them into three groups:

Lions like to both rise and go to sleep earliest of all and are renowned for being 'morning types'. They like to be up by 6am and asleep by 10pm.

Bears prefer to both rise and go to sleep slightly later, usually waking around 7am and crashing into bed around 11pm.

Wolves have the latest sleep–wake preferences; they are the night owls among us. Given the choice, they would rise at 8 or even 9am and go to bed at midnight or even 1am.

There is of course much, much more to chronotypes, as you'll discover. But I felt it was important to introduce these terms to you now – after all, they are a cornerstone of the book and pivotal to knowing exactly how best to improve your sleep.

REFLECTION TIME

Each chapter will end with a few key questions, so grab a journal or use the notes section in your phone and answer as you go along. I also want you to think about a key takeaway for yourself as you get to the end of each chapter, so keep that in mind while you're reading too. If you're open to it, I would love nothing more than for you to share your key takeaway with me (for details on how to get in touch, refer to the 'Closing notes' at the end of the book, pages 261–2).

★ Which of the seven key signs of sleep deprivation ring true to you?

★ Do you recognise any of the signs in your best friend, partner or co-workers?

★ Do you regularly wake exhausted after eight hours of sleep and if so, do you now understand why?

★ Do you feel you get sufficient SWS? Why/why not?

★ Which chronotype do you think you are and what is your best friend?

★ What's the most valuable takeaway from this chapter?

2

TAKE THE QUIZ: FIND YOUR CHRONOTYPE

I can guess, when you picked up this book and read the title, your first thought was, *Oh, I wonder which one I am – Bear, Wolf or Lion?* Or perhaps you read the previous chapter and upon learning the basics of chronotypes, you may have thought, *Well, sometimes I'm a Wolf, other times a Bear – it depends on my mood, or if it's the weekend!* Trust me, I have you covered! Time to find out what chronotype you are. Let's take the quiz. Simply write down the number, or circle it in the book, of the answer that most reflects you.

QUIZ: WHAT'S YOUR CHRONOTYPE?

What time would you like to wake up in the morning, given the choice?

1. Before 6am
2. Between 6am and 8am
3. After 8am

What time do you prefer to go to bed?

1. Before 10pm
2. Between 10pm and 12am
3. After midnight

How do you feel upon waking?

1. Fresh and full of energy
2. Dozy, but after a coffee or tea, good to go
3. Exhausted – I need a few hours to fully wake up

Compared to others, how much sleep do you need?

1. Less: I feel fine on seven or so hours
2. Around average: seven to nine hours
3. More: I could sleep for ten-plus hours

When do you find yourself most productive?

1. Before midday

2. Between 10am and 2pm

3. In the late afternoon and evening

At work, how do others most describe you?

1. A leader

2. A team player

3. A social butterfly

At work, what's your key strength?

1. Leadership, vision and strategy

2. Getting what needs to get done, done

3. Creativity and unconventional, original ideas

Do you consider yourself:

1. Future-oriented – always thinking about what's next

2. Both future- and present-oriented

3. Present-oriented

If you go out at night, how likely are you to stay out late – to 10 or 11pm?

1. Rarely – that's my bedtime

2. Sometimes, perhaps once over the weekend

3. Regularly – I love late nights

How would you characterise your overall health?
1. Good
2. Fair
3. Poor

Do you find it easy to be healthy? That is, sleep sufficiently, exercise regularly and eat well?
1. Yes – I'm renowned for it
2. Sometimes yes, sometimes no
3. Temptation usually gets the better of me

What's your biggest challenge?
1. Perfectionism
2. Saying no to others' requests
3. Sleep

Results ...

Add the numbers you have circled (or written down) to get a total. If you scored:
12 to 19 points – you are a Lion
20 to 28 points – you are a Bear
29 to 36 points – you are a Wolf

THE LION

In a nutshell, Lions like me are natural-born leaders – we are positive, proactive and goal-oriented. Our commitment to excellence and conscientiousness means we are often high achievers too. As a partner, we're stable, loyal and go above and beyond for the ones we love. With friends and family, we invest heavily in a few key relationships and are often referred to as a 'good influence'.

Your behaviours: You're early to rise and love your morning routine – it's likely to start at the gym, yoga, or with a run. With productivity peaking in the first half of the day, you like to tackle the most challenging tasks of the day first. That said, by late afternoon, you're often mentally sapped, so you find yourself retreating for some much-needed recharge time – socialising, exercising, or simply soaking up some sun. In the evening, your energy is at an all-time low, so you love nothing more than a relaxed dinner and early bedtime – after all, you want to be fresh for the morning.

At work: You are strategic, analytical and forward-thinking.

At play: You are health-oriented, risk-adverse and enjoy routine.

In a relationship: You are stable, committed and dedicated.

31

Socially: You prefer quality over quantity – think intimate experiences over large gatherings.

Biggest strength: You are a leader for proactivity and positivity – in your best light, it radiates from you.

Biggest challenges: Perfectionism and staying in the here and now – you're always thinking about what's ahead, sometimes to your detriment.

Best careers: Anything that leverages your leadership qualities – CEO, director, manager, president, producer or business owner.

Health concerns: Anxiety.

Famous Lions: Richard Branson, Oprah Winfrey, Tim Cook (Apple CEO) and Anna Wintour (editor-in-chief of *Vogue*).

THE BEAR

Grounded, level-headed, humble and reliable – if you are a bear, others can depend on you, day or night, whatever the request. Known as hard-working team player, you love to be in a group and find yourself most motivated when you're part of a team, whether for work or pleasure. As a partner, you're generous and giving and typically put the needs of your loved one before your own. This extends to your family and closest friends too.

Your behaviours: Around 7am, you begin to rise – and head straight for a coffee to clear out that brain fog. After an hour or so, and maybe coffee number two, you're ready for action. Throughout the day, mini-breaks see you through – that is, until 3pm, when, like clockwork, that slump hits. And, if you are sleep deprived, it's even worse. Come evening, you're pretty wiped out; however, you can also find it hard to switch off.

At work: You are team-oriented, industrious, humble – nothing is beneath you.

At play: You are flexible and relaxed.

In a relationship: You are dependable and easy-going.

Socially: You're friendly, caring and love to keep everyone happy.

Biggest strength: Your reliable and hard-working nature means you deliver when needed – personally and professionally.

Biggest challenges: Prioritising your own needs – often you're so busy pleasing others, you forget about yourself, which may cut into your needs for rest and relaxation.

Best careers: Anything that leverages your natural work–life balance and reliability, ranging from a primary caregiver, nurse or teacher to corporate roles with these requirements. Although you aren't driven to become a leader, this often happens naturally, simply because you're hard-working, dedicated and industrious.

Health concerns: Fatigue and depression.

Famous bears: Barack Obama, J.K. Rowling and Arianna Huffington (co-founder of the *Huffington Post* – or *HuffPost*).

THE WOLF

If you're a Wolf, you're the night owl of the chronotype world. Wolves have two sides – you can be sociable, fun-loving and invigorating, but you're also prone to sleep deprivation, which can leave you feeling stressed and anxious. At work, you're a creative soul who shines when working on a project that you're truly passionate about; however, when bored, you're easily distracted and may procrastinate. At home, you squeeze the last bit out of every day, even if it means burning the candle at both ends. Socially, you are connected to many circles, but when you're in an intimate relationship, you may withdraw and spend most, if not all, of your time with your partner.

Your behaviours: If you had your choice, mornings would start at 8 or 9am with a double-shot espresso. However, should you need to rise earlier, a sociable coffee date or breakfast is your preferred way to start the day. After a slow-ish morning, your creative juices kick into gear and you notice that the later the day gets, the more you get into your flow. If you're working on something and you're completely absorbed in it, this can continue well into the evening – even in the absence of others. However, if you do call it quits at work, you're usually keen for some adventure in the evening. You're quite energised by now, after all. That said, if you're sleep deprived, you may not be so enthusiastic about venturing out – cue couch time with Netflix. Of all chronotypes, you go to bed the latest, with lights out often creeping into the early hours of the morning. However, this doesn't bother you too much – life is to be lived, right?

At work: Creative and unconventional.

At play: Spontaneous, daring, curious – you like to explore new places, people and experiences.

In a relationship: Playful, uninhibited.

Socially: You like everyone to have a good time and you are probably the last one to leave the party.

Biggest strength: Making the most of every day.

However, if you're sleep deprived, you may be limited in your ability to do so.

Biggest challenges: Being exhausted in the morning, yet wide awake in the evening.

Best careers: Something creative – entrepreneur, writer, singer, dancer, artist, designer, inventor.

Health concerns: Insomnia, bipolar disorder.

Famous Wolves: Pharrell Williams, Jay-Z, Elon Musk and Elvis Presley.

FAQ ABOUT CHRONOTYPES

Can we change chronotypes?

One of the first things I'm asked about chronotypes is, 'Can I change it?' To that, I say – yes. Your chronotype is equally determined by internal factors (your genetics) and external factors (your environment and sleep saboteurs) – it's a fifty-fifty split. So, while you can't change your DNA, you can modify your behaviour and possibly shift chronotypes.

Another question I hear is: 'I don't resonate with some of the characteristics of my chronotype. Does that mean it's not for me?' No, this can happen! Firstly, you may be a hybrid (see below). Secondly, at best, only 80 per cent of our chronotype's 'true' nature will come through at any given time (and even less than that if you are suffering from things like stress or insomnia).

Is it possible to be two different chronotypes?

No, but you can be on the cusp of two; for example, on the cusp between a Bear and a Wolf. This is likely if your results were close to those of another chronotype:

- 19 for being a Lion on the cusp of a Bear

- 20 for being a Bear on the cusp of a Lion

- 28 for being a Bear on the cusp of a Wolf

- 29 for being a Wolf on the cusp of a Bear.

How common is each chronotype?

This is a hard question to answer; however, recent research into our sleeping habits leads me to believe that the Wolf is perhaps the most common chronotype. Initially, it was theorised that around 50 per cent of us were Bears, 25 per cent Wolves and 25 per cent Lions. However, a 2020 study in the *Journal of Sleep Research* found that 51 per cent of people suffer from clinically significant sleep problems, which is a hallmark sign of Wolves.

When and how did chronotypes originate?

Although chronotypes are a relatively new concept in mainstream media, in sleep psychology, they are decades old. Interest in them was first sparked in the 1970s by Swedish researchers: first, Professor Oscar Öquist with his thesis 'Charting Individual Daily Rhythms'; then by James A. Horne and Olov Östberg, who created the Morningness–Eveningness questionnaire (MEQ), which is still used in clinical practice today and formed the basis of the quiz in this chapter.

In 2017, chronobiology reached a new high when researchers Jeffrey Hall, Michael Rosbash and Michael Young won the Nobel Prize in Physiology and Medicine for their discoveries into the circadian rhythm, including the fact that 50 per cent of our genes (not just our sleep–wake cycle) are under circadian control.

In 2021, chronotypes research elevated to a new, never-before-seen height when Australia's leading sleep expert, Olivia Arezzolo, profiled them in her bestselling book, *Bear, Lion or Wolf* . . .

Okay, maybe that last one is still coming to fruition, but I do see it coming to life eventually – just you wait!

Where is the Dolphin?

You may have heard about the Dolphin chronotype, so this is a fair question. As I said in my introduction, I have chosen to omit a fourth chronotype because, based on my own research and experiences with my clients, I believe the Dolphin chronotype is more likely to be an extreme version of the Wolf. If you've done other sleep quizzes and been categorised as a Dolphin, read over the description of the Wolf again – my feeling is that a lot of the characteristics will resonate with you!

I'm a different chronotype to my partner and apparently our circadian rhythms don't align. Are we doomed?

Definitely not! You can be a different chronotype to your partner, or friends and family, and still get along happily. The key word here is compromise. Sure, there may be 'ideal' times to do certain activities (for example, eat, wake, sleep, have sex), but that doesn't mean you can't do them outside of these specified times. For the best results for both parties, try to meet in the middle – wherever that is.

REFLECTION TIME

★ Which chronotype are you?

★ Do the behaviours and personality traits of your chronotype resonate with you?

★ Which chronotype is your best friend and/or partner?

★ Which chronotype would you like to be, given the choice?

★ What's the biggest takeaway you have from this chapter?

3

FACTORS THAT INFLUENCE CHRONOTYPES

As you're about to discover, both inherent and environmental factors can influence our chronotypes. This is especially important to know if you're a Wolf. Although you are technically at a disadvantage when it comes to your circadian rhythm, it's helpful to know that this isn't set in stone – there are many factors you can change, allowing you to evolve beyond your current circumstances.

INHERENT FACTORS

Genetics

When you think about it, do either of your parents have the same chronotype to you? Although I've mentioned my mum is a Bear and I am a Lion, what I haven't said is that my dad is a Lion and my brother is a Bear. This is no coincidence: 50 per cent of our sleep personality is predetermined by DNA.

The most important gene for our circadian rhythm is PER3. A 2003 study published in the academic journal *Sleep* found that a longer variant of the PER3 gene results in eveningness (Wolves), whereas a shorter variant correlates with morningness (Lions).

There are several other genes that are relevant to our circadian rhythms. While we all have these genes, only some of us have these specific variants.

- The other 'Period' genes – PER1 and PER2 – some variants are associated with morningness.

- CLOCK (circadian locomotor output cycles kaput) genes, which affect the length of our circadian cycle. Depending on your CLOCK gene variant, you may have a 'short' cycle, which would then increase the likelihood of you being a Lion, or a 'long' cycle, which correlates with being a Wolf.

- RGS16 and FBXL13 genes – variants in either of these genes increase your likelihood of being a Wolf.

Your genes can also influence whether your need for sleep is high, medium or low, which can impact your chronotype. Lions generally need the least sleep, Wolves the most and Bears somewhere in between. One gene specifically related to our sleep needs is the DEC2 gene. A 2018 study by the University of California found that those with a unique variant of this gene needed only 6.25 hours of sleep to feel rested – much less than those without the gene variant, who typically needed 8.06 hours of sleep.

Another gene related to short sleep needs is the DRB1 gene, which promotes wakefulness. Those with a variant of this gene are naturally inclined to be awake for longer periods of time and sleep less. As Lions have the lowest sleep need, it's possible that if you are a Lion, you have these 'short sleep' variants.

CHRONOTYPES AND GENE VARIATIONS

Lions: may have variations in PER1, PER2, PER3, CLOCK and DEC2 genes.

Bears: may have conflicting variations; that is PER1 (predicting a Lion) and RGS16 (predicting a Wolf).

Wolves: may have variations in PER3, CLOCK, RGS16 and FBXL13.

CHRONOTYPES AND SLEEP NEED

Different chronotypes need different amounts of sleep per night to hit the refresh button. Specifically:

Lions: Your sleep need is low to medium – you can operate well on seven hours' sleep per night, sometimes even less.

Bears: Your sleep need is high – you prefer a solid eight to nine hours. If this doesn't happen, you'll probably find yourself fatigued and may rely on caffeine, sugar or alcohol to get through the day.

Wolves: Like Lions, you have a low to medium sleep need – you can easily get by on around seven hours per night. However, if you don't get this amount, you'll become sleep deprived and might find yourself needing eight hours or more.

Sensitivity to light

I'm going to harp on about light a lot because it really is our primary zeitgeber (the factor that controls your circadian rhythm). With that in mind, another critical component to consider when discussing chronotypes is light sensitivity. Just as no two people are the same, so too does light sensitivity vary from person to person.

And it can actually differ significantly – a 2019 study led by Monash University found that one person's light sensitivity can be fifty times greater than another's – fifty times! If you are highly sensitive to light, the tiniest bit of light in the evening could suppress your melatonin levels and leave you wide awake, whereas another person living with you, say your partner or housemate, could be exposed to this same light and fall asleep no problem.

Personality

Ah, personality. Whether it's determined by nature – that is, your genes – or by nurture – your environment – the fact of the matter remains: different chronotypes have particular idiosyncrasies. That said, the research here is correlational, so it's challenging to say which came first, the chronotype or the personality type. In other words, is our personality dependent on our chronotype, or is our chronotype influenced by our personality?

What we do know is that Lions are more likely to be positive, proactive and upbeat individuals, with high IQs, perfectionistic tendencies and an aversion to taking risks. They are the least likely of any profile to be neurotic or emotionally volatile, and are also least likely to suffer addictions. The more someone is morning oriented, the less likely they are to be depressed, too – though anxiety can be a problem.

Bears are typically level-headed, practical, less prone to moodiness (compared to Wolves) and balanced. They are known to be hard-working and industrious too, and often work best in groups. Of all chronotypes, they are the least likely to develop obsessive tendencies; however, they can be challenged by fatigue.

Wolves are characteristically creative, social and thrill-seeking, with an eagerness for the new. They often find it hard to concentrate and are more prone to addictions than Bears and Lions. Of all the chronotypes, Wolves are at greatest risk for insomnia, anxiety, depression and bipolar disorder and generally have the poorest health.

Age

When I was a teen, I remember coming alive in the late evenings and being eager to jump on to Myspace or MSN Messenger at that time. Now, at thirty-one, my prime rolls around at 6am, when I'm jogging, journaling or meditating. Does that sound familiar to you? Late nights were commonplace in your teens but as you get older, bedtimes become earlier and earlier? Age definitely plays a role in our circadian preferences. I will come back to this topic in more detail in the next chapter.

CHRONOTYPES AND DIFFERENT LIFE STAGES

As you've probably noticed, as we move through different life stages, our sleeping habits change. While I'll cover the reasons why this occurs in chapter four, here's an overview of the most and least common chronotype in each age group:

Infancy and early childhood

Most common: Lions

Least common: Wolves

School-age children

Most common: Bears

Least common: Wolves

Adolescence

Most common: Bears and Wolves

Least common: Lions

Adulthood

Most common: Bears and Wolves

Least common: Lions

> **Older age**
>
> Most common: Lions
>
> Least common: Wolves

ENVIRONMENTAL FACTORS

Where you live

Remember the last time you went camping and by 8pm you were out like a light? Without artificial light, we are more responsive to the day–night light patterns, which, as you may have noticed on your camping trip, means you're more likely to rise and go to sleep early (like a Lion). And the research supports this too. A 2014 study in *Chronobiology International* found that those living in rural areas (like where I grew up in Gippsland, Victoria, Australia) are more likely to be Lions.

REFLECTION TIME

★ Do you share the same chronotype to one or both of your parents? What about your siblings?

★ Have you noticed a change in your sleep–wake preferences at different life stages?

FACTORS THAT INFLUENCE CHRONOTYPES

★ Have you noticed you sleep and rise earlier when you are away from the city?

★ Which of the factors that influence chronotypes do you feel is most relevant to you?

★ What stands out to you as a key takeaway from this chapter?

4

AGE AND YOUR CHRONOTYPE

As mentioned briefly in the last chapter, as we move through different life stages, it's likely we will present as different chronotypes. I explain why this happens in more detail below.

INFANCY AND EARLY CHILDHOOD (BIRTH TO FIVE YEARS OF AGE)

FAST FACTS
- The most common chronotype among very young children is Lion (69 per cent) – the younger the child, the greater their morning preference.

- The least common chronotype in this age group is Wolf (1 per cent).

Sleep requirements per night

Birth to 3 months: 16 to 20 hours, waking every 1 to 2 hours for a feed

3 to 6 months: 14 to 17 hours – 9 to 11 hours at night and 4 to 6 hours for daytime naps

6 to 12 months: 14 to 15 hours – 9 to 11 hours at night and 2 to 3 hours for daytime naps

12 to 24 months: 13 to 15 hours – 9 to 11 hours at night and 1 to 2 hours for daytime naps

2 to 3 years: 11 to 14 hours – 9 to 11 hours at night and 1 to 2 hours for daytime naps

3 to 5 years: 10 to 14 hours at night and napping once during the day, if needed

If there's one thing for sure, it's that babies sleep . . . a *lot*! Highlighting the importance of sleep for cognitive development, a 2010 study by the University of Montreal found that babies who slept longer at twelve months had higher levels of executive functioning (including shifting attention from one task to another and self-control) at eighteen and twenty-six months. In addition, research by the University of Oxford in 2015 found that when an infant napped after learning new words, they were more likely to store the words in their vocabulary compared to infants who didn't nap.

Before they are three months old, babies don't really have a chronotype. They don't make their own melatonin, nor do they have regular circadian cycles. Rather, they obtain their sleepiness hormone from their mother's milk and sleep at all sorts of irregular times, but most particularly after a feed. However, a 2017 study in *Scientific Reports* identified that after the age of three months old, most infants – 69 per cent – have a strong morning preference (Lions, hello!), and only 1 per cent are Wolves.

Many sleeping issues at this time are caused by excessive household light – it can suppress melatonin levels by 71 per cent, leaving the little ones at risk of bedtime resistance. Although many parents feel their child is the only one unwilling to call it a night, bedtime resistance is much more common than you think. In fact, a 2013 study by the University of Colorado found that 14 per cent of infants are resistant to going to bed, as are 42 per cent of three-year-olds and 50 per cent of five-year-olds.

CHILDHOOD UNTIL ADOLESCENCE (FIVE TO ELEVEN YEARS OLD)

> **FAST FACTS**
> - Sleep requirement: nine to eleven hours.
> - The most common chronotype at five is Lion; by age seven, approximately half are Lions and Bears.
> - Wolf is the least common chronotype.

As children grow, their circadian rhythms change and many Lions morph into Bears. This is due to:

- **Biology:** As our little ones move through childhood, their circadian rhythms naturally adjust. As a result, they are more alert in the evening, sleepier in the early morning and crave a later sleep–wake time.

- **School start and finish times:** On school days, their pattern looks something like this: rise by 7am, eat, school by 9am, focus on learning until 3pm with a few breaks in between, play until 6pm, followed by dinner and relaxation time before bed. From what you know so far about sleep profiles, who does that sound like? Yep, you got it: Bear.

- **Devices:** As children grow, their eagerness for late-night activities does too. In our modern society, this often relies on technology, be it a phone/tablet, computer or television. And as you'll learn in chapter five, these blue light-emitting devices keep us up late at night and often short-change our sleep in the process. Bears are more prone to these sorts of distractions than Lions.

ADOLESCENCE (TWELVE TO NINETEEN YEARS OLD)

> **FAST FACTS**
> - Sleep requirements: nine to eleven hours per night.
> - Wolf is the most common chronotype among teens.
> - Lion is the least common chronotype.

Those teenage years of late nights! Although we like to attribute this to devices, it's not that simple. Alongside the temptations of social media and video games, there are several physiological and psychosocial changes at play here.

- **Puberty:** All mammals going through puberty experience a delay in their sleep–wake preferences, not just humans. In fact, a 2009 study in *Developmental Neuroscience* noted that this shift is so significant that if an adolescent mammal is unable to go through puberty, as in the case of castration, they do not demonstrate this circadian shift.

- **Lower sensitivity to morning light**: Teens are less sensitive to morning light, which naturally makes them sleepier in the morning. This is due to a structural change in their suprachiasmatic nucleus (SCN), a region in the brain linked with melatonin production.

- **Technology**: Of course, we can't discount the impact of tech. A 2012 study in the peer-reviewed journal *BMJ Open* found that teens using a phone in the last hour before bed are 48 per cent more likely to take longer than an hour to fall asleep and 35 per cent more likely to sleep two hours less, compared to those who don't have such late-night phone use. Both sleep-initiation difficulties and sleep inadequacy are characteristic of the Wolf.

- **Social events**: For teens, many exciting events happen in the late evening (parties and social media chatting being two primary examples). As a result, there is greater interest in staying up late and, as their brains have not fully developed, they find impulse control and self-discipline more challenging than adults do – cue staying up to the wee hours of the morning.

SLEEP DEPRIVATION IN TEENS

This is an important phenomenon to highlight. A 2006 paper by America's National Sleep Foundation found 75 per cent – yes, three in four – of teens sleep less than eight hours per night. Irrespective of the cause, this is extremely problematic. As you will recall, inadequate sleep compromises cognitive function, memory and mental health.

To manage this, a recommended strategy is to have later school or university start times. A 2017 study by Pennsylvania State University found that by starting class times after 8.30am, teens had up to 57 minutes of extra sleep per night. Furthermore, and this should be of interest to parents and governments alike, researchers at the University of Minnesota found that delaying school or university start times by just one hour can reduce teen motor vehicle accidents by as much as 70 per cent.

ADULTHOOD (TWENTY TO SIXTY-FIVE YEARS OLD)

FAST FACTS
- Sleep requirement per night: seven–nine hours.
- The most common chronotype among adults is thought to be the Bear, but, as I mentioned earlier, it's thought that the Wolf is on the rise.
- The least common chronotype is Lion.

As we emerge into adulthood, many teen Wolves become Bears. Driving this change is:

- **Conventional work hours:** Since Covid-19, I'll admit, work hours are not as traditional as they used to be. That said, many adults still work roughly between the hours of 9am to 5pm. The conventional working day echoes the structure of a school day, so it makes sense to behave like a Bear. Think about it: if we were to get up like our early bird Lion counterparts, we may run out of steam by 2 or 3pm. Or, alternatively, if we were a Wolf, we'd come into our prime in the evening and find ourselves frustrated that we weren't leveraging this perfect opportunity to work productively – something familiar to many of us, I'm sure! Thus, it makes sense to be a Bear: wake around 7am, muster up the mental energy and focus for a day of work and then rest and recuperate in the evening. And by going to bed around 11pm, we ensure we reach that golden eight hours of sleep.

- **Social psychology**: Along similar lines, it's socially conducive to be a Bear, too. By being somewhat alert in the evening after work, we can take part in social experiences, like after-work drinks, a walk or a workout. This may not be the case for Lions, whose energy levels are typically sapped by this time after rising so early.

- **Habits from schooldays**: For thirteen (or so) years, our circadian cycle was guided to wake around 7am, be productive from 9am till 3pm, then rest and recuperate for the next day. Although we may have finished school, our circadian rhythm was trained by the above schedule and, as many shift workers will know, is resistant to change.

Although Bears are still believed to be the most common chronotype, in recent years sleep issues appear to be on the rise, which is more reflective of Wolves. Some of the key sleep challenges in adulthood include:

- **Ageing:** The ageing process naturally reduces slow-wave sleep (SWS), which contributes to lighter, restless and unrefreshing sleep. A 2017 study by the University of California found that males over the age of thirty have 50 per cent less SWS and females over thirty have 25 per cent less SWS, compared to their respective counterparts in their twenties.

- **Parenthood:** While parenthood is meant to be a joy, I'm sure most new parents are not so enthused about the chronic lack of sleep. A 2018 study found that new parents attain a meagre 4.5 hours of sleep per night in the first twelve months of parenthood – yes, 4.5 hours! And even after those twelve months, on average it takes a parent around six years to fully 'recover' from the sleep lost in that first year.

Furthermore, there are significant challenges for women as they age, including:

- **PMS:** It's not your imagination, ladies, one third of menstruating women experience sleep disturbances in the weeks preceding and during menses. Specifically, during the late luteal phase (the days before a period), women spend fifteen more minutes of the night awake instead of asleep. This is due to a fluctuation in oestrogen and progesterone. They play a role in thermoregulation and, as a result, your body finds it difficult to keep cool when you're menstruating, which impairs melatonin secretion. With respect to chronotypes, all of them suffer, just at different times. Research shows Lions are the most likely to sleep poorly in the week prior to menstruation, Bears, around four days before and Wolves, in the day or two immediately before their period.

- **Pregnancy**: A bundle of joy for your heart, not so much for your sleep. As noted in the academic journal *Obstetric Medicine* in 2015, up to 94 per cent of women report sleep disturbances throughout pregnancy. This can be attributed to a number of factors, such as:

  - hormonal fluctuations – variations in hormones, such as oestrogen, can impair the stability of your core body temperature. As melatonin production relies on a cool core body temperature, this is a key reason why pregnancy can exacerbate sleeping problems.

- increased bladder pressure – waking to use the bathroom . . . again? It's only natural, as your bladder is squeezed by your growing bub, after all!

- discomfort – cramping, restless legs and backaches – pregnancy is a joy, right?! Needless to say, these can leave you tossing and turning all night, and having sub-par sleep.

- **Menopause:** After pregnancy and caregiving to our little ones, you'd hope sleep could return to what it was – right, ladies? While this is true for a period of time, once we reach menopause, we again face significant challenges. A 2020 paper by the University of Toronto reported that up to 60 per cent of post-menopausal women experience sleeping problems, compared to only 30 per cent of pre-menopausal women. This can be largely attributed to oestrogen, again. It declines at this time, impeding melatonin synthesis, necessary to initiate and maintain sleep. As mentioned above, this hormone is pivotal in keeping a cool core body temperature, needed for production of our sleepiness hormone. Another factor perpetuating sleeping issues in menopause is a dip in the hormone progesterone. Progesterone usually helps us produce gamma-aminobutyric acid (or GABA). This neurotransmitter slows the central nervous system, which helps you to feel calmer. During the day, it enables you to stay relaxed and 'switch off' when needs be; in the evening, it helps you to fall asleep, sleep deeper and wake up less through the night. A third consideration for menopausal women is depression. Research by India's KG Medical University in 2015 identified that as many as one in five menopausal women experience depression. And, as you'll learn later, depression is a risk factor for problematic sleep.

OLDER ADULTS (SIXTY-FIVE YEARS AND OVER)

FAST FACTS
- Sleep requirement: seven to eight hours.
- The most common chronotype in older adults is the Lion.
- The least common chronotype is the Wolf.

Ask your grandma to come to a dinner at 9pm and she (like I) would probably baulk at the suggestion – that's sleep time, after all! As we age, there is a notable general shift in our chronotypes. We see few, if any, Wolves, fewer Bears and many Lions. This can be attributed to:

- **Natural advancement of the circadian cycle**: Basically, the opposite of what happened in puberty; in older age, the circadian rhythm naturally shifts to an earlier sleep–wake time.

- **Fewer evening commitments**: Social psychology plays a role here: there is less reward or reason to stay up late. Long gone are the days of dancing until the wee hours of the morning; instead, late nights are (usually) preserved for much-needed rest.

- **More leisure-oriented daytime commitments**: Instead, older adults are more inclined to socialise during daylight hours – particularly once they have retired and are free of work commitments. Thus, there is an eagerness to be alert and energised for these activities, which may start in the morning. And due to the widespread sleeping issues (discussed below) faced by at least half of our older population, after a morning of fun, they can feel flat and fatigued, even at 4pm. Hence, they call it a day quite early, which is characteristic of Lions.

As mentioned, and as I'm sure you've noticed, older age is synonymous with sleeping issues. The core reasons include:

- **Ageing eye lens:** The natural ageing process yellows the eye's lens, which consequently decreases the amount of blue light entering the eye. While excess blue light can be a problem, in moderation it is actually helpful; it serves to regulate the circadian rhythm and maintain a consistent sleep–wake schedule.

- **Continued decline in (sleep preserving) hormones:** For females, ageing sees a further decline in oestrogen and progesterone and, as discussed previously in 'Menopause', this exacerbates sleeping problems. In addition, for both males and females, testosterone loss, which is a natural consequence of ageing, is a problem too – so much so that the degree of this loss can correlate with the severity of the sleeping issue.

- **Comorbid conditions:** Another reason older adults struggle to sleep properly is due to chronic illnesses. As you'll read later, many illnesses, such as depression, obesity and Alzheimer's, increase the likelihood of sleep issues.

- **Chronic pain:** My grandma suffers from arthritis and when it flares up, she is literally up all night, tossing and turning, in immense pain. Unfortunately, her experience is more common than not: a 2015 study published in the peer-reviewed journal *BMJ Open* found that 53 per cent of older adults experience chronic pain, which undoubtedly leaves many unable to sleep.

- **Medication use:** Many older adults regularly take pharmaceutical medication, something that can exacerbate sleeping problems. While this is covered in greater detail in chapter five, it deserves a mention here. In part, it explains why so many older adults suffer problematic sleep:

  - antidepressant (SSRIs) users are almost twice as likely to suffer insomnia – 17 per cent of users do, compared to 9 per cent of non-users

  - those taking pain medication, such as opioids, are 42 per cent more likely to suffer insomnia

  - users of anti-inflammatory tablets, such as aspirin, spend twice as long awake through the night compared to non-users.

- **Vitamin deficiency:** Many older adults are deficient in sleep-supportive nutrients. As noted in 2010 by the

US Institute of Medicine, 67 per cent are deficient in magnesium, 46 per cent are vitamin C deficient and 32 per cent are low in vitamin B6. As you'll read later, this is a considerable problem for sleep.

- **Napping:** According to a 2016 study in the academic journal *Sleep Medicine*, 27 per cent of those aged 65 and above nap frequently, compared to only 12 per cent of their younger counterparts. On average, nappers take 39 per cent longer to fall asleep, compared to non-nappers.

REFLECTION TIME

- ★ What life stage are you in and do the sleep patterns and challenges highlighted here resonate with you?

- ★ If you experience or have experienced sleeping issues, are they common for your age group?

- ★ Does this chapter help you understand more about your family's sleeping patterns and perhaps why family members are a particular chronotype?

- ★ What surprised you the most in this chapter?

- ★ What is one key takeaway that stood out to you?

5

SLEEP SABOTEURS

I would say most of us love a little late-night scroll on our phones or a Netflix binge, or perhaps we work later on the computer than we know we should. It's just so tempting, isn't it? You're deep in a groove and although the clock says 10pm, it feels like it's mid-afternoon and you could keep going for hours. I'll be honest: even I find disconnecting from tech challenging, but I do so because I know just how bad it is for my sleep, and even worse for my energy levels the next day.

So, with that in mind, here are your top sleep saboteurs – the factors that are making it hard for you to fall asleep and stay asleep, and therefore making you feel unrefreshed in the morning. I'm also going to share how these factors relate to your specific chronotype, which essentially answers the question: *how bad are these sleep saboteurs . . . for me?*

TOP THREE REASONS WHY YOU CAN'T FALL AND STAY ASLEEP

1. Light

Our prime zeitgeber (factor controlling the circadian rhythm) is light and it has a lot to answer for. A 2014 study by Rush University Medical Center in Chicago found that four hours of artificial (or electric) light can delay your melatonin production by more than one hour. As melatonin is critical to you falling asleep easily, this means your household lights can contribute to your sleeping difficulties. Even if you have your lights down low, research published in the journal *PNAS* in 2019 showed that a dim interior light left on overnight can impair melatonin synthesis by 50 per cent, which could be the cause of your nighttime wakings too. However, not all light is the same.

Blue light (see boxed text), stemming from screens and household lighting, is the most sleep sabotaging, particularly in the hours before sleep. However, regardless of the light source, what's important to note here is your individual sensitivity to light (as I mentioned earlier, it can vary significantly between individuals). So if you're not sure how sensitive to light you are, do your sleep a service and avoid it at all costs.

WHAT IS BLUE LIGHT?

Blue light is a specific type of light wavelength (400–500 nanometre), shown to impact sleep and alertness. Specifically, it signals to the pineal gland to suppress the sleepiness hormone melatonin, leaving you feeling alert and awake. In the daytime, this is of course an advantage. However, in the evening, it is a problem. Instead of feeling sleepy, we feel 'wired but tired' and find it difficult to fall asleep.

2. Electronic devices

According to a 2011 Sleep in America poll, around 90 per cent of US citizens are on devices in the hour before bedtime. As a result of tech use at night, many of us suffer an array of sleeping problems – inability to fall asleep or stay asleep, or sleeping lightly and waking foggy and fatigued. Plain and simple, tech is a huge sleep saboteur and this is true for all chronotypes.

For those finding it hard to fall asleep, a study published in *BMJ Open* in 2012 found that:

- using a phone in the last hour before bed increases your likelihood of taking over an hour to fall asleep by 48 per cent

- using a computer in this timeframe increases this likelihood to 52 per cent

For those finding it hard to get *enough* sleep, the same study revealed:

- using a phone in the last hour before bed increases the likelihood of losing two or more hours of sleep by 35 per cent

- using a computer in this timeframe increases this likelihood to 53 per cent.

Even if you're using a night mode setting on your device, you may still face sleep difficulties: a 2018 study by Rensselaer Polytechnic Institute in New York found that 'night mode' only lessened the negative effect of blue light on your melatonin levels by 4 per cent. Specifically, without using night mode, blue light suppressed melatonin by 23 per cent; with night mode, blue light suppressed melatonin by 19 per cent. Thus, night mode made a meagre 4 per cent difference.

So, what if computers and phones aren't your thing but the television is? Though you may be able to fall asleep with ease (I'll admit, put a movie on any time after 9pm and I'm asleep within two minutes), you probably find you wake up through the night. This isn't just you and me though – the 2012 *BMJ Open* study mentioned above identified that those watching television before bed were the most likely to report nighttime wakings.

Lastly, if you use an e-reader, you may think you're doing the right thing by avoiding television or your phone, right? Unfortunately, this is not the case: a 2018 study by sleep scientists at Brigham and Women's Hospital in Boston found that e-readers can suppress melatonin levels by 55 per cent.

Needless to say: put your devices away, Lions, Bears and Wolves alike.

While use of electronic devices can affect us all, the chronotype most likely to suffer at the hands of this sleep saboteur are Wolves, as they are more alert in the late evening and, understandably, crave stimulation at this time. Wolves are also more prone to addiction (a finding reported in 2016 by the University of Heidelberg in Germany), so they're likely to be even more susceptible to a bit of late-night scrolling and Netflix bingeing than the rest of us.

WHY ARE DEVICES ADDICTIVE?

The biological roots of addiction lie within the brain's reward pathway. Each time you receive a text, laugh at a meme, win a game or get a 'like' on your Instagram, it produces dopamine, the 'feel good' neurotransmitter. As a result, we seek out the same action that took place prior to our dopamine hit. If you are feeling stressed, then your dopamine levels are often depleted, making the pleasure gained from tech even more appealing – and addictive. Over time, this process can override the brain's frontal lobe, which is responsible for decision making and judgement. So, if you feel bad for not being able to simply 'switch off' from tech, don't blame yourself. It's your biology, and it's completely normal.

3. Stress

I'm sure this is no newsflash to any of us, but of all the reasons we can't sleep, stress is one of the biggest. This isn't a coincidence. We are biologically programmed this way. When stressed, our bodies become hyper-stimulated, pump out adrenaline and move into 'fight or flight' mode. Historically, this is what allowed our species to survive. If we were stressed by a predator, for example, the extra energy from our adrenaline hit meant we could run away faster or fight with greater tenacity to escape danger. Thus, this programming gave us an evolutionary advantage. But the key word here is 'historically'.

Today, this system doesn't serve us so well. We rarely get those temporary threats from predators; now we are stressed by modern-day pressures – and stressed chronically. Work, social commitments or keeping up with the Joneses – our stresses do not disappear, like a predator over a hill; instead they persist throughout the day and into the evening – a permanent background hum. As a result, we are now chronically hyper-stimulated, run on adrenaline and struggle to switch off – day or night.

If this resonates and you're thinking, *Well, I'm never going to be able to sleep properly, I'm always stressed!* then stay with me. I promise that there's more to come on what you – whether you're a Lion, Bear or Wolf – can do about this. For now, though, all you need to know is that stress is a major sleep saboteur and, according to research published in 2021 in the journal *Depression and Anxiety*, the chronotype most likely to suffer from stress-related complaints is Wolves.

IN TIMES OF GREAT STRESS

If you noticed your sleep quality took a dive throughout the Covid-19 pandemic, you're not alone. Insomnia became so commonplace that sleep specialists coined the term 'Covid-somnia'. As a result of ongoing stress caused by uncertainty, instability and lockdowns (to name but a few stressors), additional blue-light exposure from tech, plus a change in our routines, many of us continue to struggle with sleep even if we didn't before the pandemic.

DIET MATTERS

Being (half) Italian, I can testify that food is life! With respect to sleep, this also rings true. Sometimes, food is sleep supportive; at other times, it's sleep sabotaging.

And it's not just what we eat – how and when we eat matters too.

Late-night eating

If you've noticed late-night snacks can keep you up for hours, it's not your imagination. The closer you eat to bedtime, the longer it takes you to fall asleep. Research published in the *Journal of Clinical Sleep Medicine* in 2011 showed that participants who ate a carb-based dinner an hour before bed took 47 per cent longer to fall asleep, compared to another night when they ate that exact same meal four hours before bed.

Further to that, late-night eating can desynchronise the circadian rhythm, leaving you more fatigued in the morning. With respect to chronotypes, this is particularly concerning for Wolves. A 2013 study published in *PLOS One* found that Wolves consume around 50 per cent more calories after 8pm (either from dinner or late-night snacks) compared to Lions. So, as tempting as it can be to have a 9pm dinner with friends or indulge in some late-night chocolate, try to refrain from eating for at least around three to four hours before bedtime.

Insufficient protein

Protein is fundamental to melatonin production – tryptophan, an amino acid found in protein, is a precursor for melatonin production. As a result, if you have insufficient protein in your diet, you compromise your ability to produce melatonin and therefore may struggle with sleep. A 2016 study published in the peer-reviewed journal *Advances in Nutrition* found that low protein intake results in sleep-initiation difficulties and waking up unrefreshed. The evidence also indicated the lower the protein intake, the worse the sleep problem.

With respect to chronotypes, there is no clear correlation between how much protein you're likely to eat and your chronotype. When it comes to diet, what is probably more relevant – for Lion, Bears and Wolves alike – is whether you're a vegan or vegetarian, as, statistically speaking, your protein intake is likely to be lower than non-vegetarians.

High saturated fat intake

A cuppa with a chocolate slice, a picnic with a cheese board, butter on your bread – this is what dreams are made of, right? Not in sleep land. These foods, and others high in saturated fat – full-fat dairy, chocolate, fatty cuts of meats – actually hinder slow-wave sleep (SWS) and REM sleep, which can lead to daytime fatigue.

High sugar intake

When you're sleep deprived, resisting sugar seems almost impossible. As mentioned in chapter one, a study led by the University of Chicago in 2004 found our cravings for sugary carbs increase by 45 per cent after only two nights of insufficient sleep – let alone weeks or months of it. However, this feeds into the cycle of sleeplessness: a 2020 study led by Columbia University in New York found that individuals with the highest intake of sugar are 16 per cent more likely to suffer insomnia, compared to those with a lower intake. Any of us with insufficient sleep – whether you're a Lion, Wolf or Bear – is at risk of this sleep saboteur.

Caffeine

There's no other moment quite like that early morning sip of coffee – right? Although I drink tea, I'm 100 per cent with you on it being a sacred moment. However, as your sleep coach, I have to be the bearer of bad news: a 2013 study led by Henry Ford Hospital in Detroit indicated that caffeine can reduce sleep length by more than one hour and double the time it takes to fall asleep. This was the case when coffee was drunk one, three or even six hours before bed – so, yes, that afternoon espresso matters.

And before you say, 'I only have coffee in the morning, so I'm fine!', unfortunately, this is not the case. Research led by the University of Zurich in Switzerland in 1995 showed that two morning coffees can reduce your total sleep time, too.

Although Wolves are thought to have the highest caffeine use, a 2016 study by the University of South Australia noted that participants with poor sleep quality (which could relate to Lions, Bears and Wolves) consume 32 per cent more caffeine than participants with good sleep quality.

LET'S GET PHYSICAL

While exercise can be sleep supportive, it's a pretty hard task when you're sleep deprived and the thought of even walking to your car seems like too much effort. Unfortunately, this perpetuates a cycle of sleeplessness; inadequate movement is a risk factor for low-quality and insufficient sleep.

With respect to chronotypes, a 2011 study in the journal

Sleep identified that Wolves typically spend 27 minutes less per day engaged in physical activity compared to Lions and Bears. That said, Bears are known for low activity levels, too.

As for late-night exercise, gentle to moderate intensity (for example, a post-dinner walk) is definitely okay, but vigorous exercise at this time is not. High-intensity workouts within an hour or less of bedtime result in a rise in core body temperature, an increased heart rate and elevated cortisol levels, none of which are conducive to sleep. The chronotype at greatest risk here is Wolves, as you're naturally the most energised in the evening, so it may seem logical for you to train late. If you do feel the need to exercise after dinner, try to ensure it is only moderate in intensity and stops at least 90 minutes before bedtime; according to a study published in the *European Journal of Sport Science* in 2020, this kind of activity will not have a detrimental effect on sleep.

SUBSTANCE USE

A night cap may seem like the perfect way to nod off but trust me, it's not. That, and other illicit substances, significantly compromise your sleep.

Alcohol

Give me an Aperol spritz and I'm a happy woman. However, I keep an eye on my alcohol intake because I know what a sleep saboteur it can be. According to a 2019 study in the *Journal of Nursing Research*, 75 per cent of alcohol drinkers wake too early and 69 per cent struggle to stay asleep.

And I can almost be certain when these nighttime wakings will occur, too – at around 3 or 4am. The first reason for this is because of 'the rebound effect' – a term used to describe the spike in the hormone cortisol, which occurs after the sedative effects of the alcohol have worn off.

Alcohol consumption can also create an imbalance between slow-wave sleep (SWS) and REM sleep, resulting in more SWS and less REM sleep. This decreases overall sleep quality, which can result in shorter sleep length and more sleep disruptions.

Research in *Chronobiology International* in 2012 indicates that Wolves are likely to be higher consumers of alcohol than Lions or Bears. However, given alcohol is one of our most common coping mechanisms, all chronotypes should keep an eye on alcohol consumption in order to maximise the chances of a good night's rest.

A FEW DRINKS CAN'T HURT, RIGHT?

Unfortunately, they can. A 2018 study in *JMIR Mental Health* reported that even a low alcohol intake – two standard glasses, for instance – reduces sleep quality by 9 per cent. Moderate consumption compromises sleep quality by 24 per cent and heavy consumption lowers it by 39 per cent.

The second thought you may be having is, *What about afternoon drinks? Surely they can't affect sleep as the effect will have worn off by bedtime.* Admittedly, it is preferable to consuming alcohol right before bed, but afternoon drinks still matter – the alcohol left in your system can still suppress REM sleep and contribute to nighttime wakings.

Cigarette smoking

Though many smokers wish they could quit the habit, the fact is that if you do smoke, it's a problem for your sleep. Smokers sleep, on average, 43 minutes less, wake more frequently through the night and attain less SWS and less REM sleep. This is especially likely if you smoke in the evening, as nicotine is a stimulant, awakening the body in a similar fashion to caffeine.

And I'm sorry to say, vaping isn't any better – it's the amount of ingestion that counts.

With respect to chronotypes, a study of over 400,000 individuals by Biobank in the UK found that Wolves are twice as likely to be smokers compared to Bears, while Bears are more likely to be smokers than Lions.

Marijuana

Although they are both from the cannabis plant, CBD is something I recommend for sleep (as you'll read later), whereas marijuana is not. Research led by the University of Michigan in 2016 found that the sleep quality of participants who used marijuana daily was 48 per cent worse than non-users and sleep maintenance was a key issue. Given that marijuana suppresses both slow-wave sleep and REM sleep, these findings make sense. Wolves, given you are most susceptible to developing addictions, you are most at risk here.

Cocaine

This increasingly common party drug enables users to stay up all night, which can in turn lead to oversleeping the next night in order to repay the 'sleep debt'. As a result, cocaine can contribute to circadian misalignment and lead to more nighttime wakings.

As noted in a 2013 study by the University of Michigan, Wolves should be particularly mindful as this chronotype is the most susceptible to drug use and addiction.

OVER-THE-COUNTER AND PRESCRIPTION MEDICATIONS

While over-the-counter and prescription medications can be useful in treating a range of ailments and health concerns, some of them can also compromise sleep. Before specifying why and to what degree, please note that if this is relevant to you, speak with your health professional as to the best course of action and whether there might be any alternatives available. Definitely DO NOT simply stop taking your prescribed medications without proper medical guidance.

Pain medication (opioids such as codeine and morphine)

It's double-edged sword: can't sleep with pain, can't sleep with pain medication. A 2018 study in the journal *Sleep Health* found that insomnia is 42 per cent more likely among (chronic pain medication) opioid users, compared to non-users. With respect to chronotypes, Wolves, you are more likely to use these medications, so watch out for this sleep saboteur.

Anti-inflammatories such as aspirin

Even the humble aspirin can spell disaster for your sleep. A 2014 study led by the University of Toronto found those who took an aspirin before bed spent 20 per cent of the night awake – double that of non-users, who, on average, spent 10 per cent of the night awake. However, when we are sick, our sniffles, coughs and general aches and pains may well prevent us from falling asleep or cause us to wake during the night, so the risk of taking aspirin needs to be weighed against the possible benefits.

SLEEPING PILLS/BENZODIAZEPINES

Though sleeping pills can help you to fall and stay asleep, the issue is what happens the next day. As noted in a 2015 study published in the journal *Sleep Disorders*, a staggering 80 per cent of benzodiazepines users experienced fatigue and fogginess the day after taking them. This fatigue is so significant that health professionals call this phenomenon the 'benzo hangover'. A 2010 paper in *Psychiatric Times* highlighted that without an alternative way to sleep properly, up to 40 per cent of users take sleeping pills long term, even though most know this is not advised. This compounds the 'benzo hangover'.

With regards to chronotypes, Wolves are most likely to take psychiatric medications, which may include sleeping pills.

OCCUPATIONAL FACTORS

Working hours

Long day at the office . . . again? While this may serve your job, it definitely doesn't serve your sleep. A 2017 paper by the University of Queensland noted those working forty-plus hours per week were 65 per cent more likely to have inadequate sleep (less than seven hours a night). With Bears known to be industrious and hard-working, this may mean that many of you are suffering at the hands of this sleep saboteur. That said, Lions, you are known to be perfectionists, which could see you working longer hours than recommended.

Shift work

I know shift workers well; my Bear mum is an aged-care nurse. Due to her rotating roster, her sleep can be haphazard. And it isn't just her – a 2010 paper in the journal *Sleep Medicine Clinics* noted 75 per cent of shift workers report sleep disturbances through the night, leaving 90 per cent of them fatigued in the day. Similarly, a 2020 study by Hanyang University in Korea found shift workers are 2.5 times more likely to develop insomnia than non-shift workers.

The reason for this can be traced back to our biology. Essentially, the circadian rhythm is thousands of years old; we are pre-programmed to sleep during typical darkness hours and be alert during typical sunlight hours. For many shift workers, this is not possible. As a result, you face an uphill battle – you're literally fighting against your biology.

Wolves, I'm happy to report that this is one sleep saboteur for which you are not at the greatest risk. Due to your natural rhythms, a Wolf working nights may actually accommodate quite well; however, a Lion would most likely struggle with night work.

LET THE SUNSHINE IN

With longer work hours, more indoor leisure activities (hello, Netflix) and concerns over skin cancer, as a society we are increasingly becoming sun deprived. This is a problem for our sleep for several reasons.

First, sunlight is a natural source of vitamin D, a sleep supportive micronutrient. As noted in a 2018 study in the journal *Nutrients*, if we become deficient in vitamin D, we are 59 per cent more likely to experience poor sleep.

Second, sunlight promotes the production of serotonin, the happiness hormone. As you'll discover in later chapters, this hormone is pivotal for mental health and, as a result, also our sleep health.

Third, sunlight (particularly in the morning) resets the circadian rhythm, helping us to feel energised during the day and sleepy at night. However, many of us are opting out of early morning walks in favour of sleep-ins. As a result, we now rely on sleep-sabotaging caffeine to give us our daily kickstart, which can cause further problems down the line.

With reference to chronotypes, those who stay up late and sleep in – common for many Wolves – are most likely to miss out on that all-important morning light. However, all chronotypes living in locations with limited light (such as countries in the Northern Hemisphere in winter) may also receive insufficient sunlight and suffer from sleep difficulties as a result.

THE HABITS OF SLEEPING

Activities in bed outside of sleep

Especially on those chilly days, watching television or doing work from your bed seems like the perfect idea – I hear you! But for your sleep, this is a definite no no. Research led by King Khalid University in 2020 found that 57 per cent of those with poor sleep hygiene (which includes doing activities in bed) find it hard to fall and stay asleep. This can be attributed to 'sleep psychology': the more you reserve your bed for sleep and sleep only, the more it becomes a cue for sleepiness. On the other hand, the more non-sleep-related activities you do in bed, the more it becomes a cue for wakefulness. Wolves should especially watch out for this sleep saboteur (no late-night Netflix binges in bed!).

Sleeping in

The best way to spend the weekend, right? As much as I want to say yes, it is, the sleep coach inside of me has to say no, it's not. The problem arises when you need to go to sleep and wake up at your regular time again – on Sunday night/Monday morning, for instance. As melatonin operates on a twenty-four-hour cycle, delaying sleep one night (Saturday) so you can sleep in the next morning (Sunday) makes you resistant to bed at the regular time the next night – and even if you do go to bed, chances are, you won't be tired enough to fall asleep quickly and will lie there ruminating.

With respect to chronotypes, the weekend sleep-in is characteristic of many Wolves. A 1999 study in the *Journal of Sleep Research* found that Wolves will go to bed 60 minutes later and rise a staggering 2.3 hours later on weekends. However, the data also showed that Wolves had around twice the amount of 'sleep debt' to Lions, which might be why they crave the weekend sleep-ins in the first place.

Going to bed by 10pm (or when you're not tired)

This is something your grandma probably told you to do with the best of intentions; after all, it technically *does* correlate with spending more time in slow-wave sleep. However, if you're a Bear or a Wolf, going to bed at 10pm can be a sleep saboteur as it doesn't align with your circadian rhythm. As a result, you can enthusiastically dive into bed and try to fall asleep, only to lay there wide awake for what feels like hours. Do this over enough nights and eventually your bed will become a cue for wakefulness and you could develop bedtime anxiety.

That said, Lions, it's perfectly okay for you to go to bed by 10pm – in fact, as you'll read in chapter nine, for your chronotype I encourage it.

Napping

Ever played 'nap roulette'? That is, you go for a nap without really knowing if you'll wake up refreshed or if you'll sleep properly that night? It's not just you – research by the University of Pittsburgh in 2010 reported that nappers take 39 per cent longer to fall asleep on days they nap, compared to days they don't. For more on why napping can be a problem, see the boxed text.

With respect to chronotypes, Wolves are more likely to nap than Lions, but fatigued Bears might be inclined to nap too – and at a sleep-sabotaging time of 4 or 5pm, which is when your energy characteristically dwindles.

WHY IS NAPPING A PROBLEM?

While I do recommend early, short naps, I don't recommend late, long ones. This is because of the impact of late naps on adenosine, a naturally occurring chemical in the body. Adenosine is a neurotransmitter which acts on the central nervous system and inhibits many of the processes associated with wakefulness. Adenosine naturally builds up in the body the longer we're awake, therefore increasing our levels of sleepiness. However, adenosine levels decrease during sleep – which is why we feel more mentally alert after a nap. But this doesn't help us if we've napped late in the day – we won't have had enough time to build up sufficient adenosine to feel sleepy, come bedtime.

ISSUES IN YOUR SLEEP SANCTUARY

This section starts with the most important factor first – and surprise surprise (!), it's not your mattress.

Temperature

Ah, balmy summer nights. I remember them well from my time living in Bali. However, I also remember waking frequently on those nights, which I'm sure resonates with many of us who toss and turn during summer.

Heat and sleeplessness go hand in hand. As mentioned earlier, this can be attributed to melatonin. This 'sleep hormone' requires a cool core body temperature to be produced. Should you become too hot, melatonin synthesis declines and you may struggle to sleep. To reduce the risk of heat-related sleeplessness, try to keep your bedroom as cool as possible (invest in air conditioning or a fan) and make sure your bed coverings are light and made from natural fibres (see more on this below).

Sheets

Here's a secret that bedding marketers don't want you to know: expensive 1,000 thread count sheets are *not* advised for your best night's sleep. In fact, the density of this thread count traps heat, which, as I've mentioned above, can contribute to sleeping problems. Another factor to consider is fabric. Artificial fibres, like polyester, can contribute to overheating too. Unlike natural fibres, they don't possess thermogenic properties – the ability to absorb and dissipate heat. So, if you can, stick to sheets made from natural fibres like cotton, linen and bamboo.

Mattress

Old, saggy mattress? Get rid of it, and quickly. In 2009, researchers at Oklahoma State University found that replacing an old mattress can improve sleep quality by 55 per cent.

ENVIRONMENTAL FACTORS

Sleeping in a new environment

Perhaps due to anxiety or a loss of familiar sleep-promoting cues from your bedroom, sleeping in a new environment is a sleep saboteur too. Although, Wolves, I have some good news for you – you're not most vulnerable here. A 2020 study by South China Normal University found that early risers are seven times more likely to suffer sleep loss while travelling than those who rise later. So, Lions, be mindful of this risk when sleeping away from home.

Noise

Trying to sleep in a noisy environment is like trying to sleep with light creeping in – it's a tough ask. A 2019 study by the University of Basel in Switzerland identified that for every ten-decibel increase in noise, sleep onset was delayed by 5.6 minutes and sleep efficiency reduced by 3 per cent. Though these numbers might seem small, it's worth remembering that ten decibels are barely audible – it's the sound of breathing. In context, this means that traffic noise can increase the time taken to fall asleep by 45 minutes, whereas noise from a nearby train station can lengthen it by a whopping 56 minutes.

A full moon

Do you wake up in the middle of the night when a full moon rolls around? Me too. This can be attributed to melatonin. A 2013 study published in the journal *Current Biology* noted we produce less melatonin during a full-moon phase, reducing our slow-wave sleep length by 30 per cent. As a result, we wake up more easily through the night.

REFLECTION TIME

★ What is your biggest sleep saboteur and how does it affect you?

★ What about the biggest sleep saboteur for your partner/best friend? If they are nearby, ask them.

★ How many of the thirty sleep saboteurs are common-place for you?

★ Does this explain why you've had sleep issues in the past or now?

★ What's your biggest takeaway from this chapter?

PART 2

STRATEGIES TO GET YOUR SLEEP BACK ON TRACK

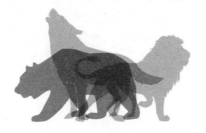

6

SLEEP STRATEGIES

One of the things my clients inevitably say is, 'I've tried everything – nothing works.' Believe me, I understand that feeling and how frustrating it is. With this in mind, I'm thrilled to share something you haven't tried: *my* science-based strategy, curated according to *your* chronotype.

Before reading this book, you may not have known that it's critical to consider your circadian cycle to optimise your sleep. It can literally make or break your results. So, keep this in mind when you're reading through these sleep strategies. Soon you will be able to apply them to your personal sleep plan for your chronotype – but more on that later.

BEDTIME ROUTINE

Having a bedtime routine is imperative. It's my go-to strategy to improve sleep. In our 24/7 society, which encourages us to go faster, do more and never rest, it's no surprise that most of us struggle to switch off at night. The reality is, without a wind-down routine before bedtime, we stay in this hyper-stimulated mode, which leaves our minds running on an endless loop with ideas and thoughts while we're trying to get to sleep.

My first recommendation for all chronotypes is to implement my signature bedtime routine. It's my signature for a reason – 100 per cent of my private clients implementing it have seen improvements in their sleep in less than seven days. It's an absolute game-changer for Lions, Bears and Wolves alike. Do note, though, that this routine is not a pick-and-choose scenario – the best results come when you do all the steps, rather than just one or two, and do them consistently, over the course of several weeks. But although there are seven steps, it can take as little as ten minutes – perfect for those who are mentally spent come bedtime (Lions and Bears, I'm looking at you!).

Signature bedtime routine

Step one: block out blue light

You may recall that light is one of the biggest factors which influences our melatonin levels; therefore, it can have the biggest impact on how easily we fall and stay asleep. In the presence of light, melatonin is suppressed, leaving you feeling alert; while in the absence of light, melatonin is produced, leaving you feeling tired and eager for bed. Outside of turning off your lights and devices each night as we've discussed, below are three ways to minimise blue light before bedtime.

- **Wear blue light glasses:** A 2018 study by Aalto University in Finland found that participants who wore 100 per cent blue light-blocking glasses (those with the distinctive red or orange lenses) before bed were able to fall asleep and wake up two hours and twelve minutes earlier. *Yes – two hours and twelve minutes!* I will add that participants in this study also had exposure to two hours of blue light in the morning, too. Wolves, with your inclination to go to bed later than you know you should, these glasses could be perfect for you.

- **Lighting:** While your devices emit blue light, so too do your household lights. As mentioned earlier, a 2014 study by Rush University Medical Center found that four hours of electric light can delay your melatonin production by more than one hour – so your household lights could well be making it harder for you to fall and stay asleep. Instead of standard lighting, I recommend red lights for evening use, with a colour temperature (which describes how 'warm' or 'cool' a light is, as seen by the human eye) below 1500k. This is particularly relevant for Wolves and on-the-cusp Bears, who are more alert in the evenings.

- **Choose a print book rather than an e-reader:** As mentioned in chapter five, e-readers can suppress melatonin levels by 55 per cent, so if you have been using one in bed, it could be the reason you struggle to fall asleep afterwards. On the other hand, a traditional book has zero effect on melatonin levels. Lions, you are the chronotype most likely to reach for a book at bedtime, so if this is the case, make sure you choose a print book.

As you can see, blocking out blue light isn't just about cutting out devices. There is so much more you can do to protect yourself, and your sleep. Wolves, as you characteristically have the poorest sleep, this step is of utmost importance for you – try to complete it at least 3 hours before bedtime. Bears, I recommend doing this 2.5 hours before bed; Lions, 2 hours.

Step two: use lavender

If bedtime anxiety is a problem, listen up. A 2010 study by the Medical University of Vienna found lavender-oil capsules could reduce anxiety by 59 per cent and improve sleep quality by 45 per cent. Similarly, a 2010 trial published in the journal *Phytomedicine* found lavender-oil capsules could reduce anxiety by 45 per cent, only 1 per cent less than benzodiazepine. Yes – just 1 per cent less than a pharmaceutical sleeping pill!

Diffusing lavender can be helpful too, as it activates the parasympathetic nervous system and helps us to feel calmer. No matter what your chronotype, lavender is perfect for those struggling to switch off and suffering anxiety.

Note: lavender is not suitable for those who are pregnant or trying to conceive, or breastfeeding. See 'complementary therapies' later in this chapter for a suitable alternative.

Step three: use a 'goodnight phone alarm'

The 'goodnight phone alarm' isn't an app – it's just the name I use for an evening alarm clock. Instead of waking you up as your morning alarm would, this one reminds you to disconnect from tech – to turn off the television, get off your laptop and stop that social media scrolling.

I'm well aware that many of us find switching off from our devices hard. Given that many apps are known to be addictive, this isn't surprising. An alarm is a great tool to support your resolve to create a healthy bedtime routine. For added benefit, label your alarm 'sleep better' – by seeing those words on your phone, you'll be reminded of your sleep goals and are more likely to follow through.

As you'll learn later in the chapter, I strongly advise a 'no tech' policy in the bedroom, so the alarm is also a great reminder to pop your phone on its charger, well away from the bedroom (out of sight, out of mind). For all chronotypes, I recommend doing this at least one hour before bedtime.

Step four: have a shower

After learning about the dangers of overheating as a sleep saboteur, it may seem counterintuitive to have a steamy shower before sleep. But, in fact, this can actually help you to cool down. When you step out of a steamy shower to a cooler bathroom, you experience a drop in core body temperature, which is a signal for melatonin production. As a result, you fall asleep more easily. While this is relevant for all chronotypes and is best done about an hour before bedtime, Lions and Bears should pay particular attention. As your energy levels typically flag at night, you may be tempted to roll straight off the couch and into bed, but a quick shower might just improve your sleep quality.

Step five: take a magnesium-based natural sleep supplement

Magnesium is the hero ingredient of most natural sleep supplements. And for good reason – it helps us to feel more relaxed. Research by the University of Leeds in 2018 found that it can reduce anxiety by 31 per cent over the course of four weeks – which makes it a great supplement for those with bedtime anxiety.

You might think you consume enough magnesium

through your diet, but in fact you may still be magnesium deficient. It's also important to note that chronic physical or mental stress depletes your body of this vital mineral.

As with any supplement, always consult your health practitioner before you start taking it.

Step six: reading or meditating

Meditating can be extremely beneficial for sleep. A 2012 paper published in *Frontiers in Neurology* found that long-term meditators have four times the amount of melatonin and spend three times longer in slow-wave sleep than those who don't meditate. Even if you're new to meditation, it's worth it for better sleep: the study showed that an evening meditation session can increase your melatonin levels, compared to nights you don't practise.

However, meditating in the evening can have a downside. Some find it anxiety provoking, while others will need to use their phone (to use a meditation app) and then may be distracted by texts or social media.

So, if meditating isn't for you, I recommend reading a traditional book – a 2009 study by the University of Sussex found reading could reduce stress by 68 per cent, with the effects beginning in just six minutes.

With regards to chronotypes, I recommend that Wolves read for at least 20 minutes to unwind before sleep, while Bears and Lions should meditate for 20 minutes.

Step seven: wear an eye mask
While we can all control our interior lighting, there are some external lights that are outside of our control – streetlights, for instance. And although these lights may be distant, they can still limit our deep sleep, leaving us fatigued upon waking. So, no matter what your chronotype, protect yourself and your shut-eye by wearing a light-blocking eye mask.

QUESTION TIME!
Write down your current bedtime routine and compare it to my signature bedtime routine.
- Which step in the signature bedtime routine are you most excited to try, and why?
- Which of these steps can you start tonight?
- What do you need to do or purchase so you can complete all of the steps?

WHAT TO DO IF YOU CAN'T FALL ASLEEP, OR YOU WAKE IN THE NIGHT AND CAN'T FALL BACK TO SLEEP

Of all problems, these are the two most common I hear from my clients. So, I've devised a five-step plan for you – Bears, Lions and Wolves alike – to help you fall asleep faster or fall *back* to sleep with greater ease.

1. If you are awake for longer than twenty minutes (either when you first try to go to sleep or after waking in the night), get out of bed and go into the lounge room

2. Put on blue light-blocking glasses

3. Diffuse lavender oil or take lavender-oil capsules

4. Read, meditate or journal

5. Only return to bed when you are just about to fall asleep

MORNING ROUTINE

While an evening routine is critical for winding down, the following morning routine is paramount to achieve good sleep too, for several reasons. Firstly, it resets your circadian rhythm, meaning you suppress melatonin earlier in the morning and produce it earlier in the evening, enabling an earlier bedtime. Secondly, as it's naturally stimulating, it reduces your reliance on things like sleep-sabotaging caffeine. While this is important for all chronotypes, those with morning fatigue – Wolves and on-the-cusp Bears – will find it the most beneficial.

1. Wake in stage 1 NREM sleep – not deep sleep

Ever woken up feeling super groggy, like you haven't slept at all – even after eight or so hours? While this could signify a lack of slow-wave sleep, it could also be 'sleep inertia' – waking up from such a deep sleep that you feel fatigued and almost drunk.

You can avoid sleep inertia by using an app or 'smart alarm clock' that detects your sleep stages and then awakens you (within a certain timeframe) in a light sleep stage. Do a search to see which ones might be compatible with your phone. Wolves and Bears, you are typically more fatigued in the mornings, so this tool might be particularly useful for you.

2. Morning meditation

If I had to tell you one thing that helps me stay calm each day, this is it. However, it's not just me – meditation literally changes our brain, gradually lowering our stress response. As a result, we feel less irritated, anxious and overwhelmed. This is the reason I recommend morning meditation for all my clients.

Ideally, you want to meditate for a minimum of ten minutes, building up to twenty minutes. If you can, meditate in sunshine (see next step). However, if ten minutes is too big of an ask, start with three, five or seven minutes – whatever is manageable. We all have to start somewhere!

Lions and Bears, take note: even if you meditated in the evening, you should still have a morning practice too.

3. Exposure to morning light

Perfect for sleepy Bears and even sleepier Wolves, this step minimises morning fatigue (hallelujah!). Quite simply, morning light suppresses melatonin and, as a result, you naturally feel more alert. Note that your circadian rhythm is the most sensitive to light in the first hour after waking, so ideally get outside then. If you get up before sunrise, or live in a location with limited morning light, the answer might be light therapy (see details later in this chapter).

4. Exercise

Just like light, exercise is another zeitgeber – it can reset your circadian rhythm. Whether it's from the release of dopamine, serotonin and endorphins, or a decrease in melatonin, the fact is that post-exercise we're naturally more alert.

Wolves, as you are typically at your most fatigued in the morning, I recommend gentle movement only – a walk is plenty. Bears, feel free to go for something a little more strenuous: think a brisk walk, light workout or yoga. Lions, you have great energy levels in the morning so can afford to go all out – a big run, sweaty aerobics class or strength training at the gym. That said, always listen to your body and adapt accordingly.

5. Limit coffee

Don't be alarmed – I said limit, not avoid! However, the word 'limit' applies to Lions and Bears here – you are advised to stick to one coffee in the morning, at specific times (as outlined in chapter nine). For Wolves, the word 'avoid' is more appropriate – particularly if you're sleep deprived and prone to anxiety. The reason is that when we're sleep deprived, caffeine has a more potent impact on our nervous system, spiking our cortisol levels. Even if caffeine doesn't usually make you anxious, if you haven't had enough sleep, this may well be a side effect. Lions and Bears, if you're lacking sleep, you should avoid caffeine too.

DAYTIME ROUTINE

Alongside avoiding sleep saboteurs like alcohol, here are five strategies to improve your sleep that you can incorporate into your daytime routine.

1. Sit by a window while you work

Simple but powerful. A 2013 study outlined in *Forbes* found workers sitting by a window slept forty-six minutes longer, compared to those working in a windowless office. The most obvious reason for this is sunlight. In addition to helping us produce serotonin, sunlight is also a key force behind vitamin D production, a nutrient important for deep sleep.

2. Wear digital readers

Digital readers are similar to the blue light-blocking glasses you might wear in the evening, but these are for daytime use. Whereas blue light-blocking glasses have red or orange lenses and block out 100 per cent of blue light, digital readers have transparent lenses and block out 40 to 50 per cent of blue light, which is ideal for the day. In appropriate amounts, blue light actually helps us to focus, be more alert and remain awake. However, in excessive amounts – as in the case for many glued to a screen – blue light can leave us hyper-aroused, anxious and feeling 'wired'.

3. Take a lunchtime walk

This is one of my all-time favourite activities. There is nothing like it for restoring a sense of calm and balance to your day. Even being away from the office or your desk for just 20 minutes can help you detach and prevent you from becoming hyper-focused and obsessive. This strategy can be particularly useful for Lions, to help keep that perfectionist streak at bay.

4. Napping

A post-lunch siesta – the perfect way to give you that much-needed second wind. Research supports this: NASA found a twenty-six-minute nap can boost alertness by 54 per cent. However, as you would have read in chapter five, napping can also be detrimental to your sleep health.

So, to save you playing another game of nap roulette, here is my perfect nap plan:

- **Keep it short – less than thirty minutes**[1]
  This keeps you in a light, stage 1 or stage 2 NREM sleep. If you nap for longer than thirty minutes, you risk entering slow-wave sleep and waking up with sleep inertia – the groggy feeling upon waking.

- **Keep it dark – wear an eye mask**
  This promotes melatonin production, optimising nap quality and depth.

- **Keep it early – start before 3.30pm**
  The specific timing will vary depending on your chronotype; however, it's best to start a nap no later than 3.30pm. This ensures there is sufficient time for adenosine to build up in the body again before bedtime.

5. Connect with nature after work

Waking through the night? If you are, Mother Nature can help. A 2019 study in *Frontiers in Psychology* found that just ten minutes spent in nature can reduce the stress

---

1 The only exception regarding nap length is for those who have slept insufficiently in the evening – perhaps shift workers or new parents. If that's you, allocate ninety minutes for your nap – you'll move through a complete sleep cycle and still wake in a light stage of sleep. However, ensure you start your nap no later than 2.30pm.

hormone cortisol. As we know, elevated cortisol levels are one of the primary reasons you wake at around 3am.

The reason for this is simple. For most people, work takes place in office buildings. As work is often a major cause of stress, over time, the office buildings themselves can become a cue for stress and elevated cortisol levels. By taking yourself out of this environment and into nature, you are allowing your body the chance to relax. In addition, fractals (repetitive patterns and shapes) that occur in nature, such as rows of trees or ocean waves, activate our parasympathetic nervous system, helping us to feel calm.

COMPLEMENTARY THERAPIES

Complementary therapies often get a bit of flack, with some arguing they don't have a scientific basis. And for some therapies, I'll agree this is true. However, the methods listed here have been verified by modern scientific research. I have personally used and recommend each of these therapies, so they come with my professional tick of approval too.

Aromatherapy

- **Lavender:** As covered in my signature bedtime routine, lavender is my go-to essential oil.

- **Orange:** If you don't like lavender, or are pregnant, breastfeeding or trying to conceive and should avoid it, orange oil is my next pick. With its calming effect on the nervous system, orange oil is perfect for anxiety-prone Lions and Wolves alike.

- **Peppermint:** Bears, your 3pm slump just got a whole lot easier. Peppermint oil has been shown to heighten alertness, fight fatigue and sharpen memory – its compound menthol stimulates the brain's neural pathways to support mental clarity. Menthol is also a natural muscle relaxant, so it may help you to feel less stressed too.

Massage

Far from being an extravagant treat, regular massage can help us get our best night's sleep, so go ahead and book yourself in. A 2013 study published in the *International Journal of Science and Research* found that, over the course of just three nights, a ten-minute back massage helped participants to both fall asleep faster and sleep more deeply. Similarly, a 2010 study in the *Journal of Depression and Anxiety* found that ten weeks of weekly massages reduced anxiety by 50 per cent. This shows that massage is ideal for anxious types, aka Wolves and Lions.

Reflexology

Another complementary therapy with promising results. A 2019 study by Shahed University in Iran found reflexology could reduce anxiety by 43 per cent and depression by 55 per cent. These two conditions, unless managed, can severely compromise sleep (for more insight into this, see 'Health Conditions Linked to Poor Sleep' in chapter thirteen). This is particularly relevant for Bears, the chronotype most likely to suffer from depression.

Acupuncture

One of my personal favourites, this traditional Chinese medicine is powerful for sleep. Research by the Omega Institute in New York in 1999 highlighted that just five sessions of acupuncture improved sleep for 94 per cent of the participants. Yes, 94 per cent!

Of all the chronotypes, Wolves enjoy new and novel experiences the most – so if you've already tried massage, give acupuncture a go.

Music or sound therapy

After recently moving into my dream home, I'll testify that the gentle echo of ocean waves crashing outside my window in Bondi Beach, Sydney, definitely helps me sleep better. It's not just me, though – a study published in *Scientific Reports* in 2017 found that playing certain sounds promoted feelings of relaxation and wellbeing among participants. And, as we know, relaxation is critical to a good night's sleep.

But which type of noise is best, you may wonder? See below for specific recommendations for your chronotype:

- White noise (for instance, a fan or static) can reduce the time it takes you to fall asleep by 38 per cent, as noted in a 2017 study by Harvard Medical School in Boston. Therefore, it's perfect for those who struggle to switch off in the evenings, which is typical of Wolves.

- Pink noise (ocean waves, rustling leaves, the human heartbeat) can increase slow wave activity (which signifies deep sleep) by 8 per cent, according to a 2017 study by Northwestern University in Illinois. As a result, pink noise is perfect for those struggling with daytime fatigue – Bears and Lions, this might be a good option for you.

- Binaural beats (which occur when you hear two tones, one in each ear, that are slightly different in frequency) have also been found to promote relaxation and therefore sleep. This therapy is ideal for Lions, who may struggle with anxiety from time to time.

My final note (pun intended) on music therapy is that you need to listen to the same sounds, beats or tunes for several weeks (at least) to see results – it gives your brain time to learn that the sounds are a cue for sleep.

OTHER THERAPIES

Light therapy

This is a great option for anyone with limited access to sunlight in the morning – for example, those living in the Northern Hemisphere during winter. A typical light therapy session involves sitting in front of a specialised device (a light therapy box or lamp) that emits bright light similar to natural sunlight. Given the influence that light has on our melatonin levels and circadian rhythm, it's no surprise that light therapy can help us to fall asleep faster and reduce morning fatigue and insomnia, as shown by a 2015 study conducted by the University of Amsterdam. In addition, light therapy can be helpful in treating depression: a 2012 study by the University of Maryland found that just one session can reduce symptoms such as morning tiredness, difficulty concentrating and general discontent. With their tendency for morning fatigue, I often recommend this therapy for Wolves, but it can be useful for all chronotypes. As always, consult your doctor or health professional before starting any treatment plan.

Cognitive behavioural therapy for insomnia (CBT-i)

If you've googled 'help me sleep better' recently, CBT-i will have come up – it's one of the most effective non-pharmacological treatments for insomnia. This therapy seeks to cognitively restructure your thoughts, beliefs and behaviours around sleep and can be initially more effective than medication, as reflected in a 2006 study by Peking University. However, researchers noted that at eight weeks, medication was shown to be more effective. That's not to say that CBT-i doesn't also work in the long term, but it takes time (often several months) and professional support to see the results.

CREATING A SLEEP SANCTUARY

One of the most common questions I am asked is, 'What should I have in my bedroom for my best night's sleep?' As you know from chapter five on sleep saboteurs, you should *not* have the following: excessive heat, devices, an old, uncomfortable mattress, high-thread count sheets or those made out of a synthetic fabric, or excess light. So, what should you do?

Keep a cool temperature

The optimal temperature for your bedroom is around 18 degrees Celsius – it reduces the likelihood of over-heating, which can impair melatonin production. This is important for all chronotypes – Wolves, statistically you have the lowest sleep quality, which suggests you may have naturally low melatonin levels; Bears, your morning fatigue will be exacerbated if you overheat during the night; Lions, your body temperature naturally rises at around 4 or 5am, so you may find yourself waking too early unless your bedroom is kept cool.

Get rid of tech

It's often tempting to check one last email or have one last scroll of social media before you go to sleep, so avoid this temptation by keeping all tech out of the bedroom (yes, this includes your phone). This is especially relevant for Wolves, who may feel more energetic and social at night.

Get the right bedding

- **Mattress:** Unfortunately, this is not a one-size-fits-all choice – it depends on your sleeping profile, body size and personal preferences. That said, replacing an old mattress – one five to ten years old – has been shown to improve sleep by 55 per cent.

- **Sheets:** Look for 200 to 400 thread count sheets in a natural fibre, such as cotton, linen, silk or bamboo, as this promotes thermoregulation and should keep your core body temperature cool.

- **Weighted blanket:** This is a therapeutic blanket that roughly weighs between 2.5 to 12 kilos. The pressure from the extra weight mimics a therapeutic technique called deep pressure stimulation, which aims to relax the nervous system. And it seems to work: a 2018 study by the University of Massachusetts found that

63 per cent of participants felt less anxious after using a weighted blanket. This blanket might be most useful for Wolves, who are prone to anxiety.

Blackout blinds or curtains

Blocking out sleep-sabotaging external lights is a must and blackout blinds or curtains can help you achieve this (along with your eye mask, of course). For the perfect sleep sanctuary, make sure the curtains fully cover the windows – even a slight slither of light can be detrimental (this goes for all chronotypes).

REFLECTION TIME

As you can see, there is a wealth of sleep strategies you can choose from. As always, before moving ahead, grab your journal or use the notes section in your phone, and answer the questions below.

- ★ Which sleep strategy are you most eager to try, and why?

- ★ Which strategies will be most helpful for you and your specific challenges?

★ Which strategies would you recommend for your best friend or partner, and why?

★ For those of you who feel as though you've tried everything, has this chapter highlighted anything you haven't tried?

★ What is your biggest takeaway from this chapter?

7

THE SLEEP DIET

Most of us tinker with our diets from time to time – be it for weight loss, health or just trying what's in vogue. While we all respect how diet impacts us physically – energy levels, skin, body composition – there's less awareness as to how it impacts our sleep. And, as you've read chapter five, you'll now know that diets low in protein, high in sugar and saturated fat, plus large, late-night dinners are all sleep saboteurs. Caffeine is another potent sleep saboteur, as is alcohol.

So now that you know what you *shouldn't* eat, I'm sure you're eager to know: what *should* I eat and does it depend on my chronotype? The truth is, there's a range of key macro- and micronutrients, which I've detailed in this chapter, that will provide the specific nutrients you need to sleep properly. In addition, I've highlighted specific superfoods and teas that can help you rest easier too.

MACRONUTRIENTS

Carbohydrates

While keto diets vilify the mere existence of carbs, you need them in order to achieve your best sleep. However, a low intake, rather than a high intake, is preferable and, unsurprisingly, complex carbs are more beneficial than simple, sugary carbs. Complex carbs have been shown to promote deep sleep, so this macronutrient is of particular importance if you are a light sleeper, or wake unrefreshed and foggy in the morning. Bears and Wolves, take note!

Sources of complex carbohydrates: whole grains, such as oats, brown rice and quinoa; legumes, such as chickpeas and lentils; vegetables, such as sweet potatoes and corn; bananas

Omega-3s

You may recall from chapter five that saturated fat is a sleep saboteur; however, *polyunsaturated* fat, like

Omega-3s, can improve sleep, as they have a special role in melatonin synthesis. Specifically, Omegas-3s minimise any abnormal fluctuations that may occur due to illness or stress, ensuring that you produce the sleepiness hormone as you should.

Sources: fatty fish, such as salmon, fresh (not canned) tuna and sardines; prawns and oysters

Vegan sources: avocado; nuts and seeds, such as walnuts, pistachios, cashews, flaxseeds and pumpkin seeds

Protein

As the building block for melatonin, protein is *the* hero sleep nutrient. A 2011 study by the University of North Dakota showed that a high protein diet can reduce nighttime wakings by as much as 21 per cent. In addition, protein – particularly the amino acid tryptophan – is vital for the production of serotonin, another important hormone for regulating the sleep–wake cycle.

Sources: poultry, such as chicken and turkey; low-fat dairy; fish; eggs

Vegan sources: whole grains, such as quinoa; legumes, such as chickpeas and lentils; soy milk and tofu; nuts and seeds

> **ISN'T RED MEAT A GOOD SOURCE OF PROTEIN?**
> Yes, it is ... however, red meat can be difficult to digest,
> creating problems with acid reflux and heartburn, which, as
> any sufferer would know, can then lead to disrupted sleep.
> In addition, red meat is often high in saturated fat, which is
> a known sleep saboteur. Fat content is also the reason I've
> specified low-fat dairy, rather than full fat.

MICRONUTRIENTS – VITAMINS

Vitamin B6

Eager to boost your melatonin levels? Load up on B6!
This vitamin helps the body to produce both melatonin
and serotonin, which directly aid sleep, plus it reduces the
risk of mental health conditions such as depression.

Finally, researchers have discovered that vitamin B6
can enhance dream recollection. So, if you're wanting
to know more about what goes on in your mind when
you're sound asleep, make sure you get your dose of B6 –
Lions, Bears and Wolves alike!

Sources: poultry, such as chicken and turkey; fatty
fish, such as salmon and fresh (not canned) tuna; low-fat
dairy, eggs

Vegan sources: soy products, such as fortified tofu; sweet potato, white potato and spinach; avocado; bananas

Vitamin B12

Another B vitamin on the sleep podium, B12 has a distinct role in regulating our sleep–wake cycle and helping your circadian rhythm maintain its normal sync. In practice, it supports melatonin to keep it running on its normal twenty-four-hour clock, enabling you to fall asleep and wake at roughly the same time each day.

Like B6, vitamin B12 also supports the production of melatonin and serotonin, so much so that those with low levels of vitamin B12 are more likely to suffer from anxiety and depression. Wolves, it's more common for you to experience circadian misalignment and mental health challenges, so please make sure you're getting your daily dose of B12.

Sources: fatty fish, such as salmon, fresh (not canned) tuna, sardines and trout; oysters; low-fat dairy

Vegan sources: if you are vegan, I recommend taking a B12 supplement; however, as always, please consult with your doctor or health professional about your individual needs

Vitamin C

Of all the vitamins and minerals, research by the University of Pennsylvania in 2015 found that vitamin C is one of the most important for sleep – even more so than magnesium and zinc. Specifically, the evidence indicated that low levels correlate with short sleep lengths (five to six hours a night).

Vitamin C also impacts mood – like several other nutrients highlighted, insufficiency is linked with depression and anxiety. As you'll read in chapter thirteen, these mental health conditions increase your likelihood of sleeping problems.

With respect to chronotypes, as Lions typically have the highest intake of fruits and vegetables, both of which are rich in vitamin C, it's unlikely they will suffer from a deficiency. On the other hand, Wolves typically have the lowest intake of these foods, which could leave you vulnerable to inadequate vitamin C intake – and shorter sleep length as a result.

Sources: most fruits, especially citrus fruits, berries, kiwifruit; most vegetables, especially leafy greens, such as spinach and kale, broccoli, Brussels sprouts, sweet potato

Vitamin D

The 'sunshine vitamin' isn't just for our bones – it's critical for optimal sleep. As mentioned in chapter five, a 2018 study in the journal *Nutrients* found those with vitamin D deficiencies were 59 per cent more likely to experience poor sleep. As vitamin D is a co-factor in serotonin and melatonin synthesis, and can activate brain regions involved in sleep regulation, these findings are not surprising.

Whether you're a Lion, Bear or Wolf, what's most important to consider is how often you are indoors – sunshine is our primary source of vitamin D. That said, there are some food sources, which I've listed below.

Sources: fatty fish, such as salmon, fresh (not canned) tuna and sardines; egg yolks

Vegan sources: mushrooms

HONORARY AWARDS

Alpha carotene: While not a nutrient in itself, the antioxidant alpha carotene, a precursor to vitamin A, deserves a mention. A 2015 study conducted by the University of Pennsylvania found that of all diet-related deficiencies linked with problems falling asleep, vitamin

---

A deficiency was number one – even more so than magnesium. As vitamin A is fundamental to eye health, this makes sense – light detected by the eye plays a critical role in regulating our sleep–wake cycle. Sources for this super-nutrient are the orange-coloured vegetables: sweet potato, carrots, pumpkin and, of course, oranges.

Lycopene: Similar to alpha carotene, lycopene is not a nutrient per se but an antioxidant protecting eye health; therefore, it plays a fundamental role in regulating our circadian rhythm. The 2015 University of Pennsylvania study mentioned above found those with a low intake of lycopene are likely to only obtain a meagre five hours of sleep a night – instead of the normal seven to eight hours – and also experience difficulties falling asleep. Lycopene is abundant in tomatoes, watermelon and papaya.

MICRONUTRIENTS – MINERALS

Calcium

You may be reading through this chapter and wonder, 'Do I really need *all* of these vitamins and minerals?' I have one answer for you: yes! With regards to calcium, the 2015 University of Pennsylvania study mentioned previously found of all sleep-supportive nutrients, it's one of the most important to help you both fall asleep and stay asleep, as it helps the brain convert tryptophan to melatonin.

Regardless of your chronotype, we all need to prioritise calcium for our best night's sleep.

Sources: fish with bones, such as salmon and sardines; low-fat dairy

Vegan sources: tofu and fortified soy milk; legumes, such as navy beans and black beans; leafy greens, especially spinach and kale; nuts and seeds, especially almonds, Brazil nuts, chia and sesame seeds

Iron

Adequate intake of this mineral is particularly important for vegans, vegetarians and menstruating women, all of whom may suffer from iron deficiencies. Low iron levels have been linked to short sleep lengths (five hours per night) – and, as we know, inadequate sleep can compound over time and cause fatigue.

In terms of chronotypes, this might be especially relevant for Lions – you typically have a higher intake of fruit and vegetables (which are mostly low in iron) than other chronotypes, so make sure you're getting enough iron from other sources. Vegan and vegetarian Bears and Wolves should also take note.

Sources: oysters; turkey; eggs

Vegan sources: legumes, such as lentils and chickpeas; soy products, such as tofu and tempeh; leafy greens, such as spinach and kale; seeds, especially pumpkin and sesame seeds

Magnesium

One of my favourite parts of the evening is to take my magnesium supplement – the feeling of relaxation that comes thirty or so minutes later is heavenly. This isn't just a placebo effect either. Magnesium helps the body produce GABA (a neurotransmitter which calms our nervous system) and inhibits the release of the stress hormone cortisol – so mentally and physically, we feel more at ease. In addition, magnesium aids melatonin production – another reason why it's so great for our sleep. Bears, Lions and Wolves, this superstar of the sleep nutrition world is for you – yes, all of you!

Sources: leafy greens, such as spinach; legumes, such as chickpeas and lentils; whole grains, such as oats, brown rice and quinoa; nuts and seeds, especially flaxseeds, hemp, chia, almonds, cashews and Brazil nuts; bananas; avocado

Selenium

If you're finding it hard to fall asleep, it may be due to a lack of selenium. Of all the vitamin and mineral deficiencies which lead to sleep-initiation difficulties, selenium is ranked in the top two. This is hardly surprising, given that low levels of selenium have also been linked to anxiety. Wolves, you typically struggle the most with falling asleep and bedtime anxiety, so get your daily dose of selenium. As you'll see from the list below, it's easier than you think.

Sources: fatty fish, such as fresh (not canned) tuna and salmon; oysters; poultry, such as chicken and turkey; low-fat dairy; eggs

Vegan sources: Brazil nuts – just one per day provides your daily recommended needs!

Zinc

This is another well-known sleep-supportive nutrient – probably because many magnesium supplements include it in their formulations. The reason behind this is simple: both minerals are utilised in the production of melatonin. In addition, like magnesium, zinc plays a role in modulating the activity of another important hormone for sleep: serotonin. With such an extensive role, it's no surprise that low levels of zinc have been linked with a lack of, and poor quality, sleep.

Wolves, be particularly mindful to load up on zinc – it will help both your sleep and your mental health.

Sources: poultry, such as chicken and turkey; low-fat dairy; oysters

Vegan sources: whole grains, such as oats, quinoa and brown rice; nuts and seeds, especially cashews, almonds, hemp and pumpkin seeds

SUPPLEMENT VERSUS FOOD SOURCES

While you can take these micronutrients in supplement form, you may be able to obtain adequate levels via your diet – both options have their advantages. Supplements mean you can generally consume a higher quantity of the nutrient, as it is more condensed. On the other hand, when consumed via a food source, the nutrient can often be more readily absorbed by the body. So, for the best results, do both: eat according to your chronotype's sleep-optimised diet and take nutritional supplements where needed. As always, before you begin any supplement regime, speak to your health practitioner first.

SLEEP SUPERFOODS

Bananas

This convenient fruit provides a multitude of sleep-supportive nutrients: magnesium, B6 and tryptophan, to name but a few. Each of these nutrients plays a role in melatonin synthesis, which is why bananas make the grade as a sleep superfood. With its innate sweetness, a banana will also keep us from reaching for other sugary, sleep-sabotaging foods. Bananas are a complex carb and provide long-lasting energy, which is why they're the perfect snack for Wolves in the morning, Bears in the mid-afternoon and Lions in the early evening.

Fatty fish, such as salmon and sardines

Not only are fatty fish like salmon and sardines packed full of sleep-friendly Omega-3s, they also deliver tryptophan and vitamin D, all of which are vital for melatonin production. A 2017 study by the University of Pennsylvania found the more fish the participants ate, the fewer their nighttime disturbances. Wolves (and Bears under stress), you typically experience the most nighttime wakings, so this is particularly relevant for you.

Legumes

Legumes (such as chickpeas, black beans, kidney beans, green peas and lentils) provide a wealth of sleep nutrients – including complex carbs, tryptophan, B6, calcium, magnesium, iron and zinc. In fact, a 2020 study by Columbia University Irving Medical Center found that a high intake of legumes helped participants to sleep deeper and wake up less throughout the night. As mentioned above, Wolves and stressed-out Bears, you typically have the most nighttime wakings, so why not load up your curries and soups with some chickpeas, lentils or kidney beans?

Kiwifruit

Packed with vitamin C and the happiness hormone serotonin, kiwifruit are another sleep superfood. A 2011 study by Taipei Medical University found sleep quality could be improved by 42 per cent after two weeks of eating two kiwifruits every night. Yes – 42 per cent! The study also highlighted a 35 per cent reduction in the time taken to fall asleep. Wolves, you are most likely to be kept awake by constant mental chatter, so grab a kiwifruit . . . or, even better, grab two!

Oats

I'll never forget the porridge my mum used to make me – or how warm, fuzzy and relaxed I felt after eating. Little did I know at the time, it wasn't just my imagination – oats contain tryptophan, complex carbs and magnesium, which together help us produce melatonin. In addition, oats provide long-lasting, stable energy, which make them the perfect food for Wolves and Bears in the morning, and Lions at lunchtime.

SLEEP DRINKS

Chamomile tea

The hero of all sleep teas, chamomile contains a compound called apigenin, which promotes relaxation. This makes it the perfect cuppa to reach for in times of stress – Lions, for you this will likely be in the early evening; Wolves, in the morning; and Bears, in the afternoon.

Green tea (regular and decaf)

Green tea … a sleep tea? Hear me out. While regular green tea does contain caffeine (around a third as much as coffee), it also contains l-theanine, a compound which helps us feel more relaxed. Like coffee, regular green tea can improve attention, focus and mental clarity, but it's unlikely to make us feel jittery, anxious or cause sleeping problems.

With this in mind, I recommend green tea, in both forms, for all chronotypes. For Wolves, one cup of regular green tea in the morning can help you fight fatigue, banish brain fog and overcome a coffee addiction. However, after you've had your one regular cup, opt for decaf – and don't drink either variety after lunch. Bears and Lions, if you've already had one cup of coffee in the morning, stick to decaf only (however, if you want to swap your morning coffee for regular green tea, that's fine – but decaf only after lunch).

Milk and honey

An oldie but a goodie, milk and honey for sleep isn't just a myth – it actually works. A 2018 study by Semnan University of Medical Sciences and Health Services in Iran found that just three days of the blend, twice a day, could help individuals sleep better. The reason for this is clear: milk contain melatonin and is also high in calcium and tryptophan, while honey helps your brain convert tryptophan to melatonin. By drinking both at once, your brain is flooded with melatonin. This makes it the ideal sleep drink for Lions, Bears and Wolves alike.

Passionflower tea

While chamomile might be the hero of all sleep teas, passionflower isn't far behind. A 2018 study conducted by Monash University in Melbourne found that drinking this tranquil tea for just seven days could improve sleep quality. This may be because of its impact on GABA, the neurotransmitter which helps us to feel more relaxed. Again, this is a great option for all chronotypes.

Tart cherry juice

A 2014 study by Pennington Biomedical Research Centre in Louisiana found that two weeks of a nightly glass of tart cherry juice (which is naturally high in melatonin) could extend sleep length by a whopping one hour and twenty-five minutes. This may be attributed to the melatonin itself, or perhaps the juice's vitamin C content – one serving provides 40 per cent of our daily needs (and, as you'll remember from earlier in the chapter, vitamin C is important to attain adequate sleep length). Bears, as you're often craving more sleep, this could be a good one for you, so drink up!

REFLECTION TIME

★ Have you ever tweaked your diet and noticed a difference in your sleep? If so, how?

★ Do you regularly consume the sleep superfoods?

★ Based on your current diet, do you feel you may lack any sleep nutrients? If the answer is yes, could you relate to the symptoms of the deficiency?

★ What is the number one takeaway for you from this chapter?

8

SLEEP SUPPLEMENTS

If there's one question I'm *always* asked, it's this: 'What sleep supplements are best?' Unfortunately, I won't be able to give you a hard and fast answer: it depends on your personal needs, health challenges, and what other supplements and medications you're currently taking. For this reason, please take this section as general advice only and consult your trusted health practitioner before starting any supplement regime.

MELATONIN

If there's one sleep supplement you may have heard about, I'm guessing it's melatonin. And rightly so – there's been a lot of research into its effectiveness in treating things like delayed sleep onset and jetlag. A study published in *PLOS Medicine* in 2018 found that, among patients with clinically diagnosed Delayed Sleep-Wake Phase Disorder (DSWD), melatonin supplements could improve sleep onset by around 34 minutes. For jetlag, a 2003 study by Liverpool John Moores University in England found that certain symptoms, such as fogginess and fatigue, could be lessened by around 50 per cent with melatonin supplements.

For Wolves, who often struggle to fall asleep, melatonin supplements might be useful in the short term. However, these are not suitable for pregnant or breastfeeding women, or people with autoimmune disorders, seizure disorders, depression, diabetes or high blood pressure. As always, seek medical advice before taking any supplements.

ADAPTOGENS

If you're overworked, overwhelmed, on the brink of burnout and sleep deprived, it may be worth considering adaptogens. As you may recall from chapter five, when we are under stress our bodies move into 'fight or flight' mode, releasing stimulating hormones such as adrenaline and cortisol (our 'stress response'). As a result, we feel more alert, awake and often anxious. If this persists over time, we feel chronically 'wired' and may struggle to sleep.

Adaptogens provide a natural 'anti-stress' buffer – they limit our production of cortisol, helping the body to 'ride out' stress. This, in turn, lessens the likelihood of anxiety, 3am wake-ups and insomnia.

There are a variety of adaptogens on offer, from CBD to reishi mushrooms. Regardless of which one you choose, it's best to rotate them over time – this prevents a tolerance building up and maximises effectivity. However, as with all supplements, it's important to speak to your health practitioner first.

CBD

After recent approval for therapeutic use in countries such as Australia and the US, interest in CBD (or cannabidiol) is growing – particularly for those with anxiety-related sleeping problems. In a 2019 study by the University of Colorado around 79 per cent of participants noted a reduction in their anxiety after using CBD, and that, importantly, this was sustained throughout the three-month testing period. Researchers in the study also found that pain could be reduced by as much as 40 per cent with CBD, suggesting that it has a relaxing effect on the nervous system.

It's important to note that CBD is not the same as marijuana, which, as we know from chapter five, is a sleep saboteur. Though both come from the cannabis plant, CBD is a non-psychoactive component and does not carry the risk of dependency. Any of the chronotypes with a chronic pain condition may benefit from CBD, but always speak to your health practitioner about the potential risks and benefits before commencing.

Reishi mushrooms

While many varieties of mushroom offer health benefits, I've singled out reishi mushrooms for a reason – they have been shown to help fight fatigue. A 2005 study by the New Zealand Institute of Natural Medicine Research found that participants who took reishi mushrooms reported a 28 per cent drop in their fatigue levels. Furthermore, they reported a 39 per cent improvement in their overall sense of wellbeing.

With respect to chronotypes, if you're a Bear, fatigue is often a common complaint, so this adaptogen may be worth trying. As always, discuss with your health practitioner first.

Ashwagandha

A respected Ayurvedic herb, ashwagandha is another powerful adaptogen for those looking to reduce stress and improve sleep. A 2012 study at Asha Hospital in India found that ashwagandha helped to lower insomnia and anxiety by a whopping 70 per cent. Similarly, a 2019 clinical trial by Patil University School of Medicine in India found that participants taking ashwagandha were able to fall asleep faster and sleep both longer and deeper. At the start of the trial, 39 per cent of the group rated their sleep as 'very poor'; by the end of the trial, only 8 per cent were in this category.

This supplement may be helpful for Bears and Wolves struggling with poor sleep. As always, speak with your health practitioner first.

PROBIOTICS

You may know that probiotics are helpful for gut health, but did you know they can be helpful for sleep, too? A 2019 study by the University of Verona in Italy revealed that after six weeks of probiotic supplements, participants reported their feelings of depression had decreased, while their sleep quality had improved by 28 per cent. This can be attributed to a several factors. First, 90 per cent of our serotonin is produced in the gut, and, as you may recall, serotonin is a precursor for melatonin. Second, a healthier gut microbiome aids absorption of sleep-supportive nutrients, like vitamin C, magnesium and zinc. And third, as reflected in the University of Verona study, by improving mental-health conditions such as depression and anxiety, sleep is indirectly improved, as well.

All chronotypes who are struggling with sleep, stress, anxiety, depression or gut problems may benefit from taking probiotics. However, not all probiotics are the same (different strains have different benefits), so make sure you speak to your health practitioner before you begin.

VITAMINS AND MINERALS

As mentioned in chapter seven, there are several vitamins and minerals that are particularly important for maintaining both good general health and good sleep. If you are struggling with poor sleep, it might be an idea to talk to your doctor about testing for deficiencies in any of the below, to see whether it's worth upping your intake from food/natural sources, or taking supplements:

- calcium

- iron
- magnesium
- Omega-3s
- protein
- selenium
- vitamin B6
- vitamin B12
- vitamin C
- vitamin D
- zinc

REFLECTION TIME

★ Which sleep supplements were recommended for your chronotype, and does this resonate with you?

★ Is there any supplement you are most eager to speak to your health practitioner about? If so, why?

★ Did you have a test for any vitamin or mineral deficiencies? If so, did the results surprise you?

★ What is your key takeaway from this chapter?

9

PERSONALISED CHRONOTYPE STRATEGIES

Lions, Bears and Wolves – this is the chapter you've all been waiting for. Now that we've covered the general strategies on how to achieve better sleep, I can share with you the juicy part: how these principles apply to *your* specific chronotype. Lions, you'll learn what to do when your energy levels flag in the evening; Bears, you'll know how to overcome that 3pm slump without needing to reach for coffee and cake; Wolves, you'll discover how to ramp up your morning energy. As I'm sure you now realise, this book isn't just about helping you *sleep* better, it's about helping you *live* better. Because that's what we're all here to do, right?

A LION'S IDEAL ROUTINE

My fellow Lion, I know you well. I know that when you're in your prime, you're the first one up and smashing through your hit list each morning. Your mental clarity is on point, you're getting up extra early to catch that 5.45am gym class and you're saying no to late-night drinks. I have no doubts you've perfected many domains in your life – business, home, pleasure, health – but a good night's sleep might be one area you want to improve.

With that in mind, I'm excited to share the following strategies with you to maximise your sleep and productivity. However, don't worry too much if you can't follow this routine perfectly all the time. I say this because you're probably an A-type high achiever and may get a little overwhelmed when things don't go to plan. Just follow the advice below as much as you can, *within reason*. I don't expect you to do this 100 per cent perfectly – and neither should you.

Your ideal chronorhythm

6am: wake up, early morning routine, exercise; this is also the best time for sex

8am: start work

10.30am: break, snack

12.30pm: lunch

4pm: finish work, snack

4–6pm: unwind time

6pm: dinner

8pm: bedtime routine starts

10pm: bedtime

Best time to:

Have sex: 6am

Exercise: 6.30am

Be productive: 8am–12pm

Consume caffeine: 11am

Drink alcohol: 2–4pm

Early morning routine and notes

6am: wake, ten minutes of meditation in morning sunlight,* journal; this is also the best time for sex

6.30am: forty-five minutes of movement – moderate to high intensity is ideal

7.30am: eat breakfast as per the Ideal 3-day diet (see later in the chapter)

---

* If morning sunlight is not available, invest in a light therapy box or lamp – see chapter six for details

8am: start work; if you're looking at a screen, use digital readers

As a fellow Lion, I know how much we love our mornings. We're typically fresh, fired up and ready to *go* in the morning. Because of this, you may want to leap out of bed and get straight to work, but a word of advice: don't. Rather, start the day taking care of your mental and physical wellbeing, with meditation, journaling and a workout. This serves two purposes: you won't feel burnt out come mid-afternoon and it also grants you an opportunity to balance your daily activities.

Finally, know that even a Lion is not going to feel on top of the world *every* single morning ... If you're sleep deprived, it's okay to take things a bit more slowly.

Daytime recommendations and notes

Recommendations:

- your productivity is peaking between 8am–12pm, so utilise this time for work

- if you work in front of a screen, wear digital readers between 8am–12pm

- enjoy your biggest meal of the day at lunchtime; also take a walk if you can

- after lunch is your best time to do collaborative work and creative projects
- set aside some 'unwind time' between 4–6pm

After your early morning routine is complete, feel free to launch into your most important work tasks straight away – after all, you're in your prime before 12pm. Mornings are the best time for challenging meetings, so schedule these accordingly.

If you drink caffeine, try to have your cup of coffee or green tea at around 11am, as this will sustain your energy throughout the afternoon (and drinking it any earlier may cause anxiety). Lunch should be your biggest meal of the day. It's also a great time to get outside in nature and take a walk – this will help to keep your workaholic, perfectionist streak at bay.

In the afternoon, you may find your energy dwindling a bit. To manage this, get outside, sit by a window or eat a healthy snack. And, if you haven't already, take off those digital readers – as we know, blue light suppresses melatonin and leaves you feeling more alert, so now is the time when blue light is a friend rather than a foe.

Lastly, make sure you have some 'unwind time' before 6pm, perhaps by doing some yoga, taking a walk or simply chilling out. By doing so, you are less likely to carry the day's stresses into the evening, which could potentially sabotage your sleep.

Evening notes

You may be feeling pretty fatigued by the evening, but it's important you don't try to rev yourself up to play with your Bear and Wolf friends – if you do, you risk throwing your circadian rhythm out of alignment and will find it harder to fall and stay asleep.

Instead, practise some self-care by curling up on the couch with a book, watching your favourite television show (with blue light-blocking glasses) or doing some gentle yoga.

If you follow the signature bedtime routine below, you'll give yourself the best chance at a great night's sleep. Know that wearing an eye mask while you sleep is *extra* important for you. As you'll probably go to bed earlier than any Bears or Wolves in your household, you want to ensure you're not disturbed by any light. Similarly, block ambient sounds with some pink noise – you'll sleep even better than you normally do.

Your signature bedtime routine

Step 1: 8pm – put on blue light-blocking glasses

Step 2: 8pm – take a lavender-oil capsule or use a diffuser

Step 3: 9pm – your goodnight phone alarm should chime, reminding you to stop using your devices

Step 4: 9pm – take a shower

Step 5: 9.30pm – take your magnesium-based sleep supplement

Step 6: 9.30pm – meditate for twenty minutes

Step 7: 10pm – turn off the light, pop on your eye mask and drift off to sleep; for an even deeper sleep, try some pink noise like crashing waves

Sleep saboteurs

Top five:

- devices
- stress
- blue light
- activities in bed
- sleeping in a new environment

While you are the chronotype least likely to sabotage your sleep, this isn't always the case. You know as well as anyone that sometimes you're guilty of finishing off work in bed, working long hours and being on your devices later than you should. Lions are also prone to bouts of anxiety, so watch out for signs of stress (such as 3am wake-ups and feeing fatigued in the morning) – as we know, stress is a major sleep saboteur. With this in mind, it's important to have healthy stress-management strategies in place – be it regular weekends away (*without* the work laptop) or a bi-weekly yoga class.

Sleep sanctuary

Top three recommendations:
- blackout blinds or curtains
- a weighted blanket (particularly if anxious)
- no devices

Of all chronotypes, you would benefit the most from blackout blinds or curtains. As your melatonin levels are typically quite low at around 4 or 5am, if any light seeps into your bedroom around this time, you may wake too early. And if you're a Lion who suffers from stress, a weighted blanket is a great addition to your bedroom – it can help you feel at ease. Finally, as for all chronotypes, it's best to keep the bedroom device-free.

Best aromatherapy

You will notice that I've recommended lavender-oil capsules or a diffuser as a crucial part of your bedtime routine. Aside from this, orange oil also promotes relaxation – so this could be a good option for you when you're working on a lengthy project.

Best sleep supplements

With your tendency to become anxious, ashwagandha could be a good option for you – it will promote feelings of calm and help you to manage stress more easily. However, note that it is best to rotate adaptogens every few months or so, so be mindful of the others that are also listed in chapter eight. A daily probiotic is key, too – as it is for all chronotypes. And, as always, please speak to your health professional before starting any supplement regime.

Best complementary therapies

As you are prone to stress and anxiety, keep this at bay with a weekly massage.

Sleep diet recommendations

Top three:

- have a smoothie for breakfast

- don't skip meals
- eat an abundance of Omega-3s

Of all the chronotypes, Lions need the least guidance when it comes to diet. That said, there are always ways to improve – which, as a Lion, I am sure you're happy to hear.

The biggest thing to consider with diet is your energy levels: high in the morning; medium in the afternoon; low in the evening. With that in mind, I recommend smoothies for breakfast – you don't want anything too heavy or it will stop you in your tracks. However, after your initial burst of energy, you'll need some protein and complex carbs in your mid-morning snack and lunch, which will help you power through your afternoon.

By around 4pm, you should load up on magnesium- and Omega-3-rich snacks, as these will help you unwind as the day draws to a close. Dinner is ideally something light and easy to digest, so it won't sap your energy levels further.

Note that it is important you don't skip meals. If you do, any anxiety symptoms you might be experiencing could become worse.

Lastly, while this three-day diet has been designed for your specific chronotype, please feel free to adapt it as you see fit. As our individual energy requirements differ, I have intentionally left out portion sizes.

Ideal three-day diet

Day One

Breakfast: smoothie with plant-based protein, banana, spinach and soy or low-fat milk

Snack: eggs or hummus on brown-rice crackers; coffee or green tea

Lunch: brown rice salad with chicken or tofu; decaf green tea

Snack: handful of nuts (choose from walnuts, almonds, Brazil nuts or pistachios) and some strawberries; chamomile tea

Dinner: baked salmon and roasted veggies

Day Two

Breakfast: smoothie with plant-based protein, banana, strawberries, chia seeds and soy or low-fat milk

Snack: low-fat ricotta and crushed almonds on wholegrain toast; coffee or green tea

Lunch: tuna and brown rice sushi with a green salad; decaf green tea

Snack: avocado on brown-rice crackers; chamomile tea

Dinner: pumpkin soup with low-fat Greek yoghurt, topped with crushed nuts

Day Three

Breakfast: smoothie with plant-based protein, banana, blueberries, chia seeds and soy or low-fat milk

Snack: low-fat Greek yoghurt with berries; coffee or green tea

Lunch: tofu, quinoa, sweet potato and almond salad; peppermint tea

Snack: banana with almond butter; chamomile tea

Dinner: grilled salmon with greens (such as spinach, kale, green beans, broccolini)

CHEERS TO TIPPLE TIME

This is relevant to all chronotypes – as you might recall from chapter five, alcohol is less than ideal for our shut-eye: it reduces sleep length and depth, and contributes to nighttime wakings, even after only a few glasses. So, while it's best to avoid alcohol completely if you're trying to improveyour sleep, if you must drink, here are the best times to do it:

Lions: 2–4pm

Bears: 3–5pm

Wolves: 4–6pm

A BEAR'S IDEAL ROUTINE

Ah, the reliable Bear. You are likely to be familiar with the trials and tribulations of sleep – or should I say sleeplessness? – including morning fatigue, the 3pm slump and bedtime anxiety.

To get through your days, you may have been riding the energy rollercoaster: up with caffeine and sugar, down with alcohol, crashing into Netflix in the evening. If this has been happening for a while, you might be nearing burnout.

But don't panic: there is a better way. The strategies I share in this section won't just help you to sleep better but *live* better. Many of my Bear clients have been in a similar boat to you. However, by adopting the routines in the following pages, they have seen real improvements in their sleep. They are able to fall asleep faster, sleep deeper and wake up more refreshed. And so can you.

Your ideal chronorhythm

7am: wake up, early morning routine; this is also a good time for sex (option 1)

8am: breakfast

9am: start work

10.30am: short break, snack

12.30pm: lunch, exercise

3pm: break, snack

5pm: finish work

5–6.30pm: unwind time

6.30pm: dinner

7pm: bedtime routine starts

9.30pm: a good time for sex (option 2)

10.30pm: bedtime

Best time to:

Have sex: 7am or 9.30pm

Consume caffeine: 8am

Be productive: 10am–2pm

Exercise: 12.30pm

Drink alcohol: 3–5pm

Early morning routine and notes

7am: wake, twenty minutes of meditation in morning

sunlight,* journal; this is also a good time for sex
7.30am: thirty minutes of movement – low to moderate intensity is ideal
8am: your earliest time for caffeine
9am: start work

While Bears typically aren't great in the mornings, if you recalibrate your morning routine, you can say goodbye to mental fogginess – really! While you won't be as peppy as Lions, you'll still feel considerably better if you make use of these energy boosters: light, meditation and mindfulness. If that seems a bit overwhelming, start small and do the most important thing first: get outside into natural light. If you are living in a location where sunlight is limited during certain times of the year, be sure to invest in a light therapy box or lamp.

With regards to exercise, keep it short – thirty minutes is plenty – and aim for something like a brisk walk or yoga.

Lastly, caffeine – I know you might be itching for one as soon as you wake up, but please hold off having your espresso or latte until at least 8am. Otherwise you risk making that 3pm slump harder than it needs to be.

---

* If morning sunlight is not available, invest in a light therapy box or lamp – see chapter six for details

Daytime recommendations and notes

Recommendations:

- do your most important tasks between 10am–2pm
- work in a team as much as possible
- take mini breaks to fight fatigue, especially in the afternoon
- wear digital readers between 1–6pm (particularly if you struggle to switch off in the evening)
- the 3pm slump is likely to come – that's okay, it's just part of you!

Daytime is when Bears shine, especially when you've had sufficient sleep the night before. You also work best in a team, so orient your day around group activities from the get-go – you'll find yourself extra motivated if you do. After all, work, exercise and your lunchtime walk will be more enticing if others are involved. Similarly, taking regular mini breaks, especially to be social, will keep your stress levels down, motivation up and lethargy at bay.

Your productivity peaks between 10am and 2pm, so if you can, organise your work day according. After all, we all know that 3pm slump is coming ... so why fight it? Instead take it as an opportunity to pause and have ten minutes of 'me time'. Get out in the sunshine, do some deep breathing or eat a healthy snack – it will give you a much-needed second wind, sans caffeine.

Stress can sometimes get the better of you – if you find yourself getting anxious, set some time aside to be in Mother Nature, whether it's simply sitting in a park or going for a walk. On that note, digital readers are a great idea in the afternoon, too – they will save you from going home feeling wired and, subsequently, being unable to sleep.

Evening notes

Evenings are a bit of a mixed bag for you, aren't they? On one hand, you're so tired all you want to do is tune out in front of the television, but when you go to bed your mind starts to race. Cue staying up late, missing out on sleep and feeling foggy in the morning.

That's why I want you to be *extra* diligent about your signature bedtime routine. Because although late-night TV feels good while we're watching it, it's one of the biggest reasons we wake through the night and find it hard to return to sleep. But if you stick to the routine – which is timed specifically for *your* needs and will see you unwind *properly* – you'll see those nighttime wakings become fewer and further between. If you do happen to wake through the night, just follow the five-step plan for falling back to sleep that I shared in chapter six.

Your signature bedtime routine

Step 1: 7pm – put on blue light-blocking glasses

Step 2: 7pm – take a lavender-oil capsule or use a diffuser

Step 3: 9.30pm – your goodnight phone alarm should chime, reminding you to stop using your devices; this is also a good time to have sex if you can

Step 4: 9.30pm – take a shower

Step 5: 10pm – take your magnesium-based sleep supplement

Step 6: 10pm – do some journaling and a twenty-minute meditation

Step 7: 10.30pm – turn off the light, pop on your eye mask and drift off to sleep; if you can, pop on some white noise like a fan – it can help you to fall asleep faster

Sleep saboteurs

Top five:

- devices
- stress
- high sugar intake

- long work hours
- physical inactivity

While stress and tech use are problematic for Bears (as they are for Lions and Wolves), what's unique for you is your 3pm slump – which may result in you reaching for a sugary treat (or two) or opting out of your post-work exercise in favour of sprawling on the couch. In addition, you may sabotage your sleep unknowingly by working long hours – after all, Bears are known for their work ethic. So, make sure you're eating healthily, keeping up with exercise and getting out of the office on time – your sleep will thank you for it!

Sleep sanctuary

Top three recommendations:
- a cool room (set that air-con to 18 degrees)
- a comfortable mattress and pillows
- no devices

If you make sure there are no devices in the bedroom, you'll eliminate the temptation to scroll through social media if you wake during the night. And although you are known to put others ahead of yourself (*'The kids need new mattresses before me – I can wait!'*), this is one time you want to put yourself first and invest in your rest. Whether it's a new mattress, comfy pillows, new sheets, or the whole kit and caboodle, you deserve to sleep well.

Best aromatherapy

Ride through that 3pm slump a little easier with peppermint oil – it can boost mental clarity and increase energy, both of which are much-needed for you by mid-afternoon.

Best sleep supplements

With your tendency to experience fatigue, I recommend reishi mushrooms. Not only can these reduce feelings of lethargy throughout the day, as an adaptogen, they can also mediate your stress response, which should reduce both bedtime anxiety and nighttime wakings. As with all chronotypes, I recommend a daily probiotic. And, as always, speak to your health professional before starting any supplement regime.

Best complementary therapies

Reflexology is a great option for you to reduce stress and improve sleep quality.

Sleep diet recommendations

Top three:

- when fatigued, opt for cooked meals
- have a hearty 3pm snack
- avoid sugary treats and chocolate

As a Bear, you love your snacks and perhaps reach for the sugar a little more than you should when sleep deprived, so this diet is particularly important for you.

Firstly, with your energy levels likely to be lacklustre on rising, I've suggested cooked breakfasts for you – raw food taxes the digestive system and we don't want to drain your already low reserves. The breakfast options are high in protein and complex carbs, which should give you the energy boost you need, without the excess caffeine.

Speaking of caffeine, I recommend just one coffee or green tea at around 8am. However, if you *really* want to give yourself the best night's sleep – and reduce afternoon fatigue – you'll leave it out altogether.

Lunch should be light – you're in your prime at this time of the day, so the last thing you want is to be weighed down by a heavy meal. However, come 3pm, you can look forward to a hearty snack. My options below are packed with protein and healthy fats, and designed to deliver lasting energy, so you can finish the day strong – without the sugary treat.

For dinner, I've suggested something quick and easy. Like your breakfast, note that your evening meal should be cooked rather than raw – after a big day, I know your body needs to rest, digestive system included. However, to ensure you don't feel too deprived, I've suggested an after-dinner treat of tart cherry juice – enjoy!

Ideal three-day diet

Day One

Breakfast: eggs on wholegrain toast with a side of spinach; coffee or green tea

Snack: smoothie with plant-based protein, banana, low-fat Greek yoghurt, chia seeds and soy or low-fat milk

Lunch: chicken, avocado and quinoa salad

Snack: low-fat ricotta and fresh berries on wholegrain toast; peppermint tea

Dinner: grilled salmon and steamed greens (such as asparagus, green beans, spinach or kale)

Snack: tart cherry juice

Day Two

Breakfast: power porridge with oats, plant-based protein and soy or low-fat milk; coffee or great tea

Snack: low-fat Greek yoghurt with fresh berries and crushed nuts; peppermint tea

Lunch: tofu, sweet potato and quinoa salad

Snack: smoothie with plant-based protein, trawberries, banana, chia seeds and soy or low-fat milk; peppermint tea

Dinner: roast chicken with roasted green veggies (such as broccoli, green beans, zucchini, kale)

Snack: tart cherry juice

Day Three

Breakfast: omelette with mushrooms on wholegrain toast; coffee or green tea

Snack: banana with almond butter; peppermint tea

Lunch: salmon salad with brown rice

Snack: avocado and tomato on wholegrain toast; decaf green tea

Dinner: chicken and sweet potato curry

Snack: tart cherry juice

LET'S TALK ABOUT SEX, BABY ...

Sex can stimulate us and it can also relax us – which is why I highly recommend it as a great activity for Bears, Lions and Wolves alike. Not only does an orgasm release feel-good chemicals such as oxytocin and dopamine, it also lowers cortisol – and these things combined can reduce our stress levels and help us to sleep better. While these effects are universal, you may have noticed that I've recommended sex at different times of the day for different chronotypes. Why? Because by following your chronotype's natural energy levels, these are the times you are most likely to orgasm. However, please don't be restricted by this – feel free to have sex outside of these times, or simply when it suits you and your partner best!

Lions: With your sex drive peaking as soon as you wake, start the day with a bit of nookie – you'll orgasm easier.

Bears: You have two options. Like Lions, sex in the morning will start your day off right – that morning fatigue will disappear quick smart. On the other hand, sex in the evening will help you to fall asleep faster. So, take your pick as to what serves you and your partner best.

> **Wolves:** With your energy levels peaking in the evening, and given your difficulties with 'switching off', the best time for you to have sex is in the evening, right before sleep.

A WOLF'S IDEAL ROUTINE

Wolves, it's time to get excited. Of any of the chrono-types, I know you're likely to be suffering the most from poor sleep, lack of energy and reduced motivation. You may have gotten into the habit of staying up late and then, when you do go to bed, struggling to fall asleep – and this may have been going on for *years*. But don't worry – help is at hand. The strategies in the following section – which have been designed specifically for your needs – will help you say goodbye to fatigue, anxiety and chronic lack of sleep.

If you fully invest in the techniques for better sleep, it will benefit you personally, professionally and in your closest relationships. Soon it will become second nature and the signature bedtime routine won't seem like a chore – you will look forward to it.

Your ideal chronorhythm

7.30am: wake up, early morning routine

8.30–9.30am: unwind time

9.30am: start work (if you can, start at 10am or even later)

11am: break, brunch

1.30pm: lunch, break

4.30pm: break, snack

5.30pm: finish work (if needs be, finish later)

6pm: exercise

6.30pm: dinner

8pm: bedtime routine starts, unwind time, snack

10pm: best time for sex

11pm: bedtime

Best time to:

Consume caffeine: ideally never, but if you must, 8.30am

Be productive: 2–6pm, sometimes later

Drink alcohol: 4–6pm

Exercise: 6–7pm

Have sex: 9–10pm

Early morning routine and notes

7.30am: wake, sit in front of a light therapy box or lamp

8am: twenty minutes of meditation, walk and a stretch
8.30am: snack, regular or decaf green tea – NO coffee!
9.30am: start work

Wolves, I'll give it to you straight: your circadian rhythm does not align with being overly alert in the morning. But at this point in your life, I'm sure you're aware of that and have been doing a good job of managing it. But with this new early morning routine, you'll handle it even better. If you invest in light therapy – which I'm sure will become your new favourite therapy – you will learn what it feels like to be naturally energised in the morning and tired in the evening. I know it sounds too good to be true, but I've seen it happen for others, so I know it can happen for you.

You may have noticed that I've included an hour of unwind time for you in the early morning, whereas the other chronotypes have it in the afternoon. While I realise this might not be possible *every* day, if it is, embrace it. And always be gentle with yourself first thing in the morning – with exercise, eating and expectations alike.

Lastly, know that you have an energy lifeline: regular (caffeinated) green tea. Use it when it's most needed, as I know this will give you the boost you need – without you having to resort to its sleep-sabotaging cousin, coffee.

Daytime recommendations and notes

Recommendations:

- do your easiest tasks first
- if possible, start and finish work later; 12–8pm would be ideal
- your peak productivity comes between 1–6pm (often even later)
- wear digital readers when feeling anxious, regardless of the time
- end the day with a workout

While your fatigue has worn off a bit by late morning, mornings still aren't your strong suit. Adapt your schedule accordingly. Ease into the day by doing the easy tasks first and, if possible, shift your working hours back. While I know later start and end times would be ideal for you, I'm also aware that we don't always get what we want, so sometimes we just have to make the best of it.

And, in fact, there are *many* ways you can naturally fight your morning fatigue – with sunshine, snacks and a few strategically timed meetings, such as one over brunch. If you can organise your day like this, you'll breeze into the afternoon feeling well rested and ready to tackle your to-do list with gusto.

Speaking of the afternoon, you'll notice that you come into your own at around 1 or 2pm, so try to leverage this – it's your time to shine. That said, I know that when you're sleep deprived, your energy levels might be quite unstable, which can easily cause anxiety. If this is the case, take a break to unwind and, if you're looking at a screen, pop on digital readers.

Lastly, with energy levels riding high at around 6pm, it's a great time for a workout.

Evening notes

While you may be tempted to work late into the evening, please don't – especially if what you've got on for the next day means you have to be up at around 7am. Even if your work doesn't involve staring at a screen, it can still stimulate you and make it harder to fall asleep – and that's the last thing we want.

Speaking of sleep, I know you may think I'm being a little over the top in the routine below by suggesting both blue light-blocking glasses and red lights, especially a whole three hours before bed, but make no mistake, it will make a big difference to your sleep. Essentially, I want you to have the best possible chance to fall asleep with ease at around 11pm.

Lastly, if you haven't fallen asleep twenty minutes after hitting the pillow, get up rather than tossing and turning. If you follow the steps described in chapter six, you will fall back asleep more quickly.

Signature bedtime routine

Step 1: 8pm – put on blue light-blocking glasses, use red night lights only

Step 2: 8pm – take a lavender-oil capsule or use a diffuser

Step 3: 10pm – your goodnight phone alarm should chime, reminding you to stop using your devices; this is also a good time to have sex if you can

Step 4: 10pm – take a shower

Step 5: 10.30pm – take your magnesium-based sleep supplement (also melatonin if you are using it)

Step 6: 10.30pm – journal and read for twenty minutes

Step 7: 11pm – turn off the light, pop on your eye mask and drift off to sleep; if you can, pop on some white noise like a fan – it can help you to fall asleep faster

Sleep saboteurs

Top five:

- devices
- stress

- alcohol
- sleeping in
- late-night eating

Wolves, you are the chronotype most likely to have your circadian rhythm out of alignment, so it's natural that many of the sleep saboteurs are particularly tempting for you. For example, you might be inclined to work late (on a blue-light-emitting screen) or do a late-night workout – all perfectly reasonable when you've got as much late-night energy as you do. However, while I can understand the reasons, it doesn't change the fact that these are potent sleep saboteurs and contributing to your sleeping problems.

Other key factors to highlight for you: stress, which unfortunately may be partly brought on by your poor sleep; alcohol, which you may be using in the evenings to help you wind down; and sleeping in, which is hardly surprising if you're sleep deprived.

Last, but not least, is late-night eating. Given that you probably feel most like socialising in the evening, this is understandable – but make sure it doesn't happen too often otherwise it will compromise your sleep.

Sleep sanctuary

Top three recommendations:

- no devices
- a weighted blanket
- blackout blinds or curtains

Wolves, when it comes to your sleep sanctuary, it's worth putting in extra effort. Give yourself the best chance of a peaceful, uninterrupted sleep by following *as many* of my recommendations in chapter six as you can – leave no stone unturned. However, there are three recommendations which will be particularly helpful for you: no devices, a weighted blanket and blackout blinds or curtains. As you know by now, devices are no one's friend when it comes to sleep; a weighted blanket is great for those suffering from anxiety (which is common for Wolves); and blackout blinds are a godsend – the last thing you want is to be woken by a pesky light just as you're nodding off.

Best aromatherapy

Lavender is the best bet for Wolves: it's a powerful oil for reducing anxiety and promoting sleep, and it's a natural pain reliever too. In addition, you might want to try diffusing peppermint oil, especially in the morning – the aroma can help with reducing fatigue.

Best sleep supplements

Like all chronotypes, I recommend a daily probiotic for Wolves. If you are particularly struggling with lack of sleep, then both melatonin and CBD might be helpful options for you. However, please don't start taking any supplements until you have sought the advice of a trusted health professional.

Best complementary therapies

Acupuncture and massage are two ideal therapies for you – they can aid with both anxiety and sleep.

Sleep diet recommendations

Top three:
- eat a snack upon rising, then your 'breakfast' at brunch time
- eat an abundance of Omega-3s and magnesium-rich foods
- avoid eating late

Wolves, you are in for a treat – this diet will help you correct your two biggest sleep issues: being extremely tired in the morning and 'wired' in the evening. Other common concerns for Wolves are anxiety, stress and depression – but with the super nutrients I've recommended on your plate, these symptoms should lessen. Last, but not least, this diet should see you sleeping longer and more deeply throughout the night.

First things first, in the morning you should take it easy – start the day with a snack, then ease into a proper breakfast at brunch time. Brunch should be a decent meal, filled with the nutrients you need – like complex carbs – to start your day right and boost those energy levels. After brunch, enjoy a sleep-friendly snack before a late lunch filled with protein, Omega-3s and magnesium.

Finally, aim to share an early-ish dinner with your Bear and Lion friends – meet somewhere between your ideal dinner time and theirs. Not only will this mean you're eating at a sleep-friendly time, by socialising you'll also ease any evening anxiety that may crop up. After dinner, you can look forward to a special snack. As with the other chronotypes, feel free to adapt the diet and portion sizes according to your needs.

Ideal three-day diet

Day One

Snack: banana with almond butter; decaf or regular green tea

Brunch: mushroom omelette on wholegrain toast; peppermint tea

Snack: low-fat ricotta on brown-rice crackers

Late lunch: chicken, sweet potato and baby spinach salad; peppermint tea

Snack: handful of Brazil nuts

Dinner: grilled salmon with steamed greens (such as asparagus, green beans, spinach or kale); chamomile tea

Snack: tart cherry juice, 2 x kiwifruit

Day Two

Snack: low-fat Greek yoghurt with berries; decaf or regular green tea

Brunch: eggs on wholegrain toast with a side of spinach; peppermint tea

Snack: smoothie with plant-based protein, banana, strawberries, chia seeds and soy or low-fat milk

Late lunch: wholegrain wrap with turkey, cottage cheese and salad

Snack: brown-rice crackers with avocado
Dinner: grilled tuna with white-bean puree and steamed greens (such as asparagus, green beans, spinach or kale); chamomile tea
Snack: tart cherry juice, 2 x kiwifruit

Day Three

Snack: wholegrain toast with nut butter; decaf or regular green tea
Brunch: overnight oats with berries and soy or low-fat milk; peppermint tea
Snack: smoothie with plant-based protein, banana, blueberries, low-fat Greek yohgurt and soy or low-fat milk
Late lunch: chickpea, avocado and quinoa salad
Snack: tuna and brown rice sushi
Dinner: tofu and sweet potato curry, topped with cashews; chamomile tea
Snack: tart cherry juice, 2 x kiwifruit

10

SUSTAINING SLEEP SUCCESS

Let's be frank: how often have you read a book or listened to a podcast, been really invigorated, told yourself, 'I'm really going to do this!' and then never *actually* followed through? If you're anything like me, many, many times. Generally, we are inspired at the start, excited to see the results we are promised, get a few days or a few weeks in and then . . . something happens. We get distracted. The weekend comes around, or perhaps a holiday. Or maybe we get busy at work and think we just don't have the time for it.

If this is you, know that this is a perfectly normal reaction. Having the strategy is only one element of change. Another is having a system in place – as in: how are you going to make and sustain these changes? And lastly, and this one is of the utmost importance, the third key component is support.

You can have a great strategy but fail to see long-term results because you lack the correct system or support, or both. In fact, have you ever considered what the right system is? Have you ever wondered why others can seem to make massive shifts in their lives, yet you struggle with seemingly simple changes – like going to bed an hour earlier?

We all guilt ourselves into believing there is a problem with us: 'I'm just not good at making change', or 'I'm terrible at forming habits – I'm too stuck in my old ways'. Another one is that we believe we are 'too busy' or that it's 'just not the right time'. To anyone who has had these thoughts, know that: a) now *is* the right time, and b) you're actually great at making change, you do it all the time.

But don't let me tell you – read on and you will see it for yourself. Based on behaviour change principles, this chapter will show you how to turn ideas into action and, ultimately, see lasting results. With respect to sleep, this may be executing your bedtime routine and finding it easier to fall asleep, waking up less often through the night or sleeping deeper. With respect to your days, it may mean greater mental clarity, productivity and less stress. Ideally, it will mean all of these things.

Remember, this isn't *just* about your sleeping life. This is about your waking one, too.

PRINCIPLES OF POWER

They say mindset is everything. Without the right mindset, when you're trying to tackle your sleep, or any problem, you're going to face an uphill battle. Thus, before asking you to take action and create lasting change, I want to get you into the right headspace. Based on my personal learnings and practices, and inspired by bestselling self-development books such as Stephen Covey's *The 7 Habits of Highly Effective People* and newer titles like Simon Sinek's *Start With Why*, I want to share with you what I believe to be the fundamentals of the 'right' headspace. While I could go on for hours about this (personal development books are my favourite, after all), to keep it short and sharp, I've summarised the five most important principles.

Before you read through them, know that I set out every day trying to adopt these in my life, but that doesn't *always* eventuate. I'm not perfect and I don't expect you to be either. However, we can *aim* to execute them as much as possible and, by doing so, the process allows us to evolve into the best versions of ourselves – sleep and life included.

Principle 1: Take responsibility for your actions

Before we can create change, we need to get one thing straight: we are responsible for our own lives. Even if you're a busy parent, an overworked professional or an impulse-prone adolescent Wolf, you need to have certainty that it is you – no one else – in control of your life.

That's not to say that external forces don't influence us, or that we are able to control everything, but we do need to be cognisant of the fundamental fact that we are responsible for our own lives. Remember:

- It's you who says yes to following your implementation intentions (more on that soon!)

- It's you who says yes to another project at work

- It's you who prioritises self-care in the evening over a night out

- And it's you who acts with integrity and allows your actions to speak louder than words.

These are your choices, your actions, your inactions. No one else can do the work for you. While I can guide, support and care for you, at the end of the day, you need to be responsible. And I mean that in the essence of the word:

response-*able* = able to make a response.

As the old saying goes: we will be judged by what we do, not what we say.

Principle 2: Realise you're a change-making master

If you've ever told yourself you're not good at making change, that you simply 'can't' form new habits or that you 'suck' at sticking at things long term, you are wrong. In fact, I bet I can help you identify countless changes you've been able to make and, subsequently, numerous goals you've been able to achieve.

For instance, when you've had a health problem and been advised to move more, drink less alcohol or even just take daily medication, did you do this, even to a small extent? Or perhaps you started a relationship and your new partner loves an afternoon walk. Have you been able to follow their lead and prioritise that on a regular basis, instead of your former behaviour? And for those who think they can't stick at something long term – ever had a job you really, really didn't like but somehow hung in there because you had to?

While the above scenarios may apply to just a few of us, I know one thing that applies to all of us. Before the Covid-19 pandemic, had you ever imagined that you would have to make such significant shifts in your lifestyle? To be honest, most of us probably didn't know it was even possible. If you had asked me if I thought I would have survived (with sanity remaining) if you took away the gym, my favourite Aperol spritz bars, the freedom to see my friends and the ability to travel overseas for the better part of two years, I would have told you: 'No way!'

Many people experienced changes beyond their wildest imaginations: home-schooling children, not going to the office, being restricted to one hour of 'outside time' a day for four essential reasons only. By comparison, the changes to my life were minor. But we all faced challenges we hadn't ever considered and got through them. If there is any proof that we can, and will, make change when necessary, Covid-19 is it.

I am certain if we took a deep dive into your past, we'd find many, many more examples of how you made changes and stuck to them. Take the quiz …

QUIZ: AM I REALLY A CHANGE-MAKING MASTER?

What difficult, yet important changes have you been able to make in your personal, professional and social life in the past month? Write them down.

Personal: _____

Professional: _____

Social: _____

What has been the benefit of doing so on each occasion?

Personal: _____

Professional: _____

Social: _____

What are your three biggest achievements to date?

One: _____

Two: _____

Three: _____

- How did they change your life?
- How do or did they make you feel?
- What changes did you need to commit to in order to see them eventuate?

> - What did you do when you wanted to give up and throw in the towel?
> - Can you do the same or similar now, to create the changes you want to see in your sleeping habits?

Principle 3: Know your 'why'

Leadership guru Simon Sinek is *all* about knowing your why – and so am I. I honestly believe knowing *why* we are doing something is as important, if not more so, than knowing the *how*. For me, this factor is at the core of what's driven me to overcome significant limitations – anxiety, depression and anorexia to name a few – to evolve into the person I am today and be here, with you, sharing my sleep strategies.

Knowing your why isn't just about you, either (that's Principle 4). The most igniting and inspiring why is actually about others – be it your partner, family, friends, colleagues or the community at large. Deep down, we all want to have a positive impact on those around us. And when we connect our current actions to this deep desire, we are motivated to act. The greater the impact, the greater the motivation and, ultimately, the more you will persist through the pain that often accompanies change.

Even sleeping better is not *just* about you. You want to sleep better so you are a more energised, enthusiastic partner and friend, a more present and productive worker and a calmer and more centred member of your community. You want to be the best version of you not just for you, but so others can experience that version of you. With that in mind, let's find your why ...

> ## QUIZ: FIND YOUR WHY
>
> Think forward. Imagine twenty-eight days into the future and you are getting the sleep you know you need because of the changes you've made in your life. How do you think this will impact:
>
> - Your physical health – and, as a result, what are you able to do with greater ease?
> - Your mental health – and, as a result, what impact will this have on those around you?
> - Your intimate relationship, family and/or closest friends – and how does this change how you 'show up' each day?
> - Specific activities that are now more enjoyable for you, and, if so, which ones and how?

- Your work:
  - what do your colleagues now say about you –
    as in, what's changed?
  - how does this improve your interactions with your
    clients?
  - has your work quality changed and, if so, how?
- What specific events or experiences would be more
  enjoyable if you were sleeping as well as you'd like?

In this quiz you will have identified a multitude of reasons
– as in, your *why*'s – to make change. If you had to single
out one from that list that will inspire you to take action
now, what would it be?

What I do is write down the answers in my journal and
revisit these questions over and over again. This becomes
my reminder of my why – and my why may change over
time. I also write down a core value of the day, something
I intend to execute. This reminds me of my why and my
ideal self (Principle 4).

Answer the 'let's imagine' questions above for what
you think might happen in three months' time, too.
With a longer timeframe, you will see more progressive,
substantial shifts – really, imagine that!

Principle 4: Be guided by your best self

I'll be honest: change isn't always easy. Even if we know our why and feel uber motivated, it can be tough at the best of times, let alone when you feel like the universe is conspiring against you. Think about it: you plan for a quiet Friday night, gear yourself up for your bedtime routine and even book in for an early morning gym class on Saturday. Then you're leaving work and your best friend texts you: 'Come and have a drink, just one.' The devil on your shoulder says, 'Go for it!' But the angel on the other shoulder says (more quietly), 'Go home!' Conflict! Sound familiar?

While I am going to give you ways to overcome this problem in the first place, when in a moment of crisis, at a crossroads or facing a conflict, simply ask yourself: what would my ideal self do? If you're not sure who that person is or what they would do, take the quiz below. Essentially, the more you can familiarise, understand and appreciate who you are in your best self, the easier it is to act in these moments of truth.

QUIZ: MY IDEAL VERSION OF ME

- In three months, I am the ideal version of myself: who am I? Alternatively, ask yourself, 'What would my partner or best friend say if I was to ask them, "Who is the ideal me?"'
- How do I feel on a daily basis?
- What do I do the same, and why?
- What do I do differently, and why?
- What are my core values?
- How do I execute each of these on a day-to-day basis?
- What action(s) can I take today that move me towards this version of ideal myself?

Principle 5: The time is now

If you're waiting for a 'better time' to create change and start living the life you really want, I'll tell you: it won't come. Think about your three biggest accomplishments, as you outlined in the quiz in Principle 2. Did you feel you were ready? Did it feel like the perfect time? Were all your ducks in a row and was everything sailing smoothly? Hell, no!

I know from personal experience that you're never going

to feel ready or that you have all the resources you need: it just doesn't work like that. And again, from personal experience, I know that one of my biggest wishes for my younger self is that I stopped waiting for that time. Instead, I would tell her: 'Olivia, stop thinking and start doing. The time is now, the moment is here, your day is today. Push your boundaries, get comfortable with discomfort and evolve into that ideal self you know you can be.'

In the absence of being able to turn back time and tell myself this, I'm telling it to you.

JOURNAL PROMPTS

You may recall that I suggested times for journaling in your personalised chronotype strategies in chapter nine. As someone who has written in a journal for years, I know the benefits of reflecting – whether it's in the morning (Lions), evening (Wolves), or both (Bears). With the aim of helping you to be reflective, grounded and grateful each day, I have created the following prompts. Feel free to use only some or all of these – whatever suits you best.

How am I feeling?: Before anything, just check in with yourself. Whatever comes up, it's okay. Your feelings are not you, they are simply extensions of you.

A highlight from yesterday: Again, connect this to how you are feeling – what helped you feel great, if anything?

A lowlight from yesterday: What was the downpoint – that moment of frustration, the time you yelled at your kids or the dog – what happened? Again, it's okay. It doesn't change the fact that it happened but it does change the likelihood of it happening again.

A lesson: Link your lesson to your lowlight – this step has stopped me from being the 'hamster on a wheel' repeating the same mistakes day after day.

Three gratitudes: Keep it simple – a beautiful conversation, a great meal, waking up feeling refreshed. Try to reinforce things within your locus of control when you can, too – it means that if you need to create the goodness again, you can.

A value of the day: As you identified in Principle 4, you have a host of values you'd like to execute. However, it can be tricky to keep *all* of them in mind, so just pick one and visualise how you will bring this into fruition.

An affirmation of the day: What do you need to hear today? If you need some ideas, here's my top ten affirmations:

- Everything is unfolding exactly as it should.

- Trust is my superpower.
- Growth is a daily choice.
- Today, I choose love.
- My most important job is to be happy.
- Everything is revealed at the perfect time.
- I am safe and supported.
- I am loved more than I will ever know.
- Today, self-care is my priority.
- My time is now.

THE SIX-STEP SYSTEM FOR CHANGE

While the principles are great overarching rules to create lasting change, and ultimately become the happiest, healthiest and best-rested version of yourself, they aren't overly practical. They don't tell you how to do what you need to do, nor do they show you how to stop doing the things you know you shouldn't. That's where this comes in: a blueprint of behaviour change.

This framework lessens the reliance on willpower, which, as you know, can sway from time to time, depending on your mood and the circumstances. Instead, it makes change a streamlined, simple process and makes it easy to move towards the future you want – in this case, that's better sleep. Whether your challenge is getting started and following through or maintaining results long term, this system is for you. I won't take all the credit for these steps though: many of these processes stem from James Clear's *Atomic Habits* – a must read.

Step 1: Have an implementation intention

Once you have read through your personalised plan, I want you to ask yourself for each action:

- What do I need to do, specifically?
- When will I do that?
- Where will I do it?

Rather than just having an action plan that sounds something like: '7pm, put on blue light-blocking glasses', give yourself greater clarity:

- I will do (behaviour X)
- at (time and place Z)
- in (location Y)

It's more tangible and you'll see roadblocks before they appear – as well as having the capacity to overcome them before they derail you. The statement is referred to as an 'implementation intention' and needs to be written for each step of your new routines.

Step 2: Make things easy

When writing your implementation intentions, first examine your current patterns and see how your new habits most easily fit. For example, if you know that at 7pm every night you are finishing up dinner, it is logistically easier to keep your blue light glasses in the kitchen, next to the sink, and have a reminder on your phone at 7pm to put them on, than it would be to have your glasses tucked away in a drawer, in your bedroom, with no alarm. Don't rely on willpower. Use tech automations, such as alarms, and cues from existing habits to help you instil the new routines. It's more likely that you'll stick at it if you do.

Then make the new habit desirable. If you're going to find it *really, really* hard to switch off the television when your goodnight phone alarm goes off then the trick is to find an alternative behaviour you love just as much – meditating, reading or having quality time with your partner. Things we love but never seem to find the time for. In a similar vein, know that weekends are going to be a sore spot for you – less drinking, early nights . . . I mean, where's the fun? I get it. I've been there. Again, make the new habit *desirable*. Early nights are appealing when you know you're getting up for a morning walk with your best friend or heading off for a romantic getaway with your partner.

Finally, surround yourself with positive influences; as in, make things socially easy. If you know your friends are bar hopping every Friday night without fail, ask them to do a brunch on the weekend instead, for example. While you can attend the Friday night frivolities, it will require you to hold strong to your willpower up against the forces of your boozy best friends. It will be hard to follow through, to say the least. With this in mind, choose your social battles and know it's perfectly okay to say no. Remember, when we are acting with our ideal selves in mind (Principle 4), sometimes this may conflict with commitments – whether personal or social – we have made. This means that, sometimes, you may need to step away from what you were doing in order to do the things you are meant to do – and become the person you want to be in the process.

Step 3: Track it

The single greatest tool I have implemented recently is habit tracking. I was inspired by a client of mine,

Hugh,* who tracked everything from his caffeine intake and bedtime, through to his 'meditation minutes' and productivity hours, and also by the book *Atomic Habits*. Habit tracking is exactly what you think it is: you track your habits. Rather than make it a clinical spreadsheet, if you're creative, like me, get nostalgic by using coloured A4 paper and pens.

Write down the new habits you're committing to as per your implementation intentions and each time you do one, you get a star. Over time, you'll see patterns. For example, on a Friday night, you may notice you always forget your nightly magnesium sleep supplement. Maybe that is because you always go out for dinner and then stay at your partner's place. Whatever shows up, know it's completely okay. It doesn't change the fact that it's happening, rather it creates awareness of it. Further, it serves to help you identify and overcome your challenges.

On a final note, a fundamental of this step is to track it daily. This will hold you accountable to make change there and then, and it gives you a little dopamine hit every time you get a star.

---

* Note: names of clients have been changed to protect their privacy

Habit tracker example for Wolves' signature bedtime routine

	S	M	T	W	T	F	S
8pm: put on blue light-blocking glasses in lounge room							
8pm: take lavender oil capsules and apply lavender in lounge room							
10pm: goodnight phone alarm goes off, stop using tech							
10pm: take a shower							
10.30pm: take magnesium-based sleep supplement in the kitchen (and possibly melatonin)							
10.30pm: read for 20 minutes in bed, complete evening journaling							
11pm: put on my eye mask and turn out the lights							

Step 4: Work towards a tangible reward

Tracking is great, as are stars, but deep down what we really want is a reward. As in, a larger, more tangible reward. While feeling good is an internal reward, as it's abstract and subject to change with your mood, in a moment of crisis, you may find yourself easily swayed by temptation. To combat this, a concrete, real-time reward for your hard work is more encouraging and will lessen the chances of us falling off track.

Get seven stars: go for dinner or get your favourite dinner delivered.

Get twenty-eight stars: order an at-home masseuse or buy yourself that new shirt you've been eyeing up.

Whatever appeals to you as a reward is completely fine – unless that reward conflicts with your ultimate goal that your habits are building towards. For example, the reward of 'staying up all night with my friends' conflicts with the goal of sleeping better, so it's not suitable. Second to that, make sure you're highly specific in what you're working towards and when you reach your desired target, honour your word.

I recommend having segmented targets: seven days, one month, six months and one year. Imagine if you managed to do your bedtime routine for 365 days? Gamechanger.

And make sure your efforts are acknowledged and appreciated by the most important person in your life: you.

Step 5: Have an accountability partner

Research from NASA found that having a scheduled check in with an accountability partner (AP) makes you 95 per cent more likely to achieve your goals. Yep – 95 per cent. Having a buddy along for the evolution is critical. Not only does it remind you that someone will be checking in on you – reminding you to take daily action – it is also pivotal to overcoming roadblocks and, ultimately, staying on track long term.

Think about it: if your boss set you a yearly target but didn't ever check in on how you were going or ask if you needed any extra support, how likely are you to get there? While you may reach your target, I can assure you it would be a lot messier and ad hoc than if you had a weekly progress report, without a doubt. Though this isn't a business target, the concept of external accountability is still valid and will make all the difference.

In terms of who should be your AP, you have options. Me, or someone like me, another coach, is the ideal scenario, as it's our role to help you reflect. In the absence of either, a close friend or family member can be helpful too; however, as it's not their place to serve you exclusively (unlike a coach), their capacity to be a sounding board and offer advice accordingly may be limited, which is perfectly reasonable.

Regardless of who you engage, you and your AP should meet once a week to discuss your progress in the first four weeks and at least fortnightly beyond this. Based on my own sessions, I have found this to be the optimal format: welcomes, highlights, lowlights, lessons, review on daily actionables, progression for the coming period. As you can see, this is distinctly different from a general catch up where chit-chat is the mood, hence why I fundamentally believe a coach is your best bet.

ACCOUNTING FOR YOURSELF

Let's pull together some of the information in this section, so you can see the why, when and where.

- Write out your chronotype's bedtime routine so each step reflects an implementation intention.
- How will you 'make it easy'?
- What will your reward be for each milestone – seven days, twenty-eight days, three months, six months, one year?

- Who will your accountability partner be? What time and day will you meet, and how often? Where will this take place?
- What will be your next habit to build when you've mastered the bedtime routine? Hint: it's in your twenty-eight-day sleep challengein the next chapter!

Step 6: Obey the principle of progression

Let's say you manage to stick to your bedtime routine week after week and you're getting seven out of seven stars on your chart. Firstly, well done! Second, what's next? As humans, we are accustomed to growth – in our relationships, career and, of course, ourselves. Whether you realise it or not, growth is at the core of our being: it's what we strive for, in all aspects of our lives.

On the other hand, if you've ever felt like a hamster on a wheel, experiencing the same day, month on month, year on year, this is simply a sign that you're yearning for growth. As we've seen, mastering sleep is a goal that can be broken into habits, such as your bedtime routine, morning routine and adopting a sleep diet. However, as I'm sure you've established, this is a lot to take on at once, so you need to respect the principle of progression and 'habit stacking' (as in, start with one habit and add on as you can).

As you'll see from the twenty-eight-day plan I've outlined for you below, each week challenges you to push a little further, bend a little more and expand yourself. It's definitely *not* the same week experienced for four weeks in a row – that would be, plainly and simply, boring. Rather, this provides a framework that accommodates the principle of progression and will see you excited and engaged over the month.

Keep in mind that this timeframe is short compared to the length of time that many of you have had sleep problems. In addition, don't expect it to be a smooth-sailing, linear elevation. I'll be frank: it just won't happen. Rather, some weeks will be great and other times, you'll feel like there are a multitude of reasons for you *not* to be sleeping – work is busy; it's your best friend's birthday and you have overcommitted to a round of social events. I expect this to happen so should you.

Just because you don't see optimal results each night *doesn't* mean you've gone backwards. It doesn't mean you should stop, give up, throw in the towel and believe yourself doomed for all eternity. Rather, what it means is that you're human and embracing the peaks and troughs that come with life in itself. In addition, it also means you need to have a good chat with your AP (accountability partner) to get back on track.

Progression isn't about things going perfectly. It's about overcoming the challenges that will undoubtedly come and staying true to your vision – which, as a reminder, is to become the best version of yourself, with the support of sleep.

REFLECTION TIME

★ With this system in mind, can you see why it's been hard for you to reach your goals in the past?

★ What steps from the above have you included in the past, if any?

★ What steps have you omitted, if any?

★ What has been the effect? If you have missed many steps, go through step by step and outline the consequences.

★ Can you see how using these steps will change your success?

★ What is your key takeaway from this chapter?

11

TWENTY-EIGHT-DAY SLEEP CHALLENGE

Bears, Lions, Wolves; this is the moment of truth. As much as I've loved to educate and empower you, my true purpose here is to inspire action. I believe that knowledge is power but *applied* knowledge is the ultimate power. That's the secret sauce, where the magic lies and the thing that will produce what you want: results.

So far, we've discussed your personalised plan, 'the five principles of power' and 'the six-step system for change'; and now, we're going to dive into the 'twenty-eight-day sleep challenge'. With a specific and reasonably short timeframe, we can leverage your current motivation into a framework that spans a month, rather than days.

And then, when you see your progress each week and start seeing the results, you'll be even more motivated to continue.

When you think about it, what's one month in your life, anyway?

You'll have twelve of them this year; and, over the space of a lifetime, close to 873 (based on 2021 life expectancy rates). So really, one month . . . it's a drop in the ocean, a tiny piece of the puzzle, a small piece of the pie. But, knowing we humans have a small attention span, I trust it's the perfect amount of time.

These next twenty-eight days are going to be life-changing, to say the least. Remember: this is your time to shine, your time to evolve, your time to become your best self.

WEEK ONE

Week One is one of the best weeks – it's when you'll notice subtle differences in your sleep, energy and mood. It's when you'll start to fall asleep more easily and wake up feeling a little less foggy. It's when you'll start to feel that little bit more human again.

However, I don't want to lead you up a garden path:

this will only happen if you follow the plan. So, without further ado:

1. On Day One, check in with yourself and your accountability partner (use the baseline report and session planner below).

2. Stock up on the sleep supports you need and get rid of household sleep saboteurs (see 'prep time', below).

3. Change up your sleep sanctuary (see breakout box).

4. Practise your chronotype's full bedtime routine for five days.

5. Practise your (chronotype dependent) ten- to twenty-minute morning meditation in light (sunlight or use your light therapy box) for at least five days.

6. Start taking your sleep supplements, after consulting your health practitioner.

Baseline report

So that you can track your progress and see quantifiable change, let's check where you're at now. Be 100 per cent honest here – there is no judgement, no right or wrong; it's just where you're at, wherever that may be. So, without further ado, answer all of the questions below with reference to the past fortnight.

1. On a scale of 1 to 10, with 10 being the best, rate your:

- sleep quality overall
- ability to fall asleep with ease
- ability to return to sleep, should you wake through the night
- feelings of refreshment upon waking
- energy through the day
- stress and anxiety overall
- stress and anxiety related to sleep
- mental clarity
- memory
- concentration
- motivation at work
- motivation outside of work
- ability to be present with others

2. Specify the following:

- how long it takes you to fall asleep
- how many times you wake through the night
- sleep length
- sleep depth
- one word to describe your sleep

3. Write down your primary goal for the week a head with respect to sleep and note how this will this impact you:

- mentally
- physically
- at work
- in your relationships

Accountability partner session planner

- Share your reflections above.
- After you've read through the action plan for the week ahead, do you perceive any roadblocks or limitations?
- If so, how can you overcome this? Map it out.
- For your AP to ask: If there is *one* thing I can do to support you this week, what is it?

Prep time!

Change up your sleep sanctuary

- Check if your mattress/pillows are truly comfortable (or if you are just putting up with them).
- Change your duvet cover and sheets – ensure the new ones are made from natural fibres and that the sheets have a 200 to 400 thread count.

- Install blackout blinds or curtains (especially for shift workers).

- Order a weighted blanket (especially for anxious Bears, Lions and Wolves).

- Set the temperature to 18 degrees Celsius on your air con if it's warmer than this in your bedroom. If you need to, get a fan.

- Take all devices out of your bedroom – phone included.

- Find alternative places for any activities you were previously doing in bed.

- Make sure your phone is plugged into its charger in another room.

- If you can, switch your bedroom furniture around (see boxed text).

CHANGE YOUR SLEEP SANCTUARY

An imperative in Week One is to change your bedroom as much as possible – I'm talking sheets, duvet cover, removing any tech, even reconfiguring the layout – it's all helpful. Why? It scrambles your cues.

If you've been sleeping poorly, the mere sight of your bedroom objects elicits a neural response of stress and

> anxiety. Thus, changing these objects is ideal because you'll have no existing association that your 'new bedroom' is connected with sleeplessness. Furthermore, it reinforces your new path – one of sleeping well, resting properly and waking up refreshed.

Clear out and restock the kitchen

To clear out:

- white sugar
- refined sugary treats you usually have for snack time (chocolate/cakes/cookies, I'm looking at you!)
- coffee (or hide it *very* well)
- pre-workout supplements
- weight loss supplements (typically contain caffeine)

To keep/buy – pantry and fridge/freezer:

This 'sleep superfoods' shopping list should cater for the sleep diets of all chronotypes, as described in chapter nine. However, in lieu of getting everything on the list below, just buy the specific ingredients you need for *your* chronotype's three-day diet to start:

- nuts – walnuts, almonds, Brazils, pistachios, cashews

- nut butter
- seeds – flax, chia, hemp
- soy products – milk, tofu, tempeh, miso
- beans – black, white, red, butter, navy
- pulses – lentils, chickpeas
- whole grains – quinoa, brown rice, oats
- tea – chamomile, passionflower, green (regular and decaf), peppermint
- stevia (as an alternative to sugar)
- fruits – bananas, kiwifruits, avocados, tomatoes, strawberries, raspberries, blueberries
- vegetables – broccoli, zucchini, asparagus, peas, green beans, spinach, kale, sweet potato, mushrooms
- fish – salmon, tuna
- poultry – chicken, turkey
- low-fat dairy – milk, Greek yoghurt, ricotta cheese, cottage cheese
- eggs
- plant-based protein powder

To buy – supplements (chronotype dependent)
- tart cherry juice
- probiotics
- magnesium-based sleep supplement

- Omega-3 oil
- CBD
- ashwagandha
- reishi mushrooms

Order sleep kit

Make sure you have what you need on hand for your chronotypes routines, such as:

- blue light-blocking devices – blue light-blocking glasses, red night lights (for Wolves, especially)
- lavender capsules
- lavender oil, especially if you are anxious or wake through the night (Lions and Wolves!)
- natural magnesium-based sleep supplement
- a printed book
- sleep mask
- a light therapy box or lamp
- digital readers
- orange oil
- peppermint oil
- calming teas

Create your habit tracker

If you haven't already, see the previous chapter and create one. You need to create this for each habit you are tracking and each actionable you are required to take.

See – just a *little* bit of prep! Once that is complete, give yourself a pat on the back – you're on track!

WEEK TWO

Start the week with some self-reflection. Check in with where you're at, celebrate the wins, assess the limitations and, importantly, learn and grow from the week that has passed. I know this process works because it's exactly what I do with my clients and, time after time, I see it grants them the introspection they need to elevate higher each week. However, in the initial period of change, it's important to know you're supported – hence why you need a weekly AP session to steer you to your best success.

1. Complete your weekly progress report (see breakout box)

2. If you have reached your targets as per your

incentive scheme on your habit tracker, reward yourself accordingly

3. Have your AP session, as per the outline above

4. Continue practising your chronotypes full bedtime routine for five days

5. Continue taking sleep supplements

WEEKLY PROGRESS REPORT FOR WEEKS TWO, THREE AND FOUR

Answer the questions with reference to the past week.

On a scale of 1 to 10, with 10 being the best, rate your:

- sleep quality overall
- ability to fall asleep with ease
- ability to return to sleep, should you wake through the night
- feelings of refreshment upon waking
- energy through the day
- stress and anxiety overall
- stress and anxiety related to sleep
- mental clarity
- memory
- concentration

- motivation at work
- motivation outside of work
- ability to be present with others

Specify the following:
- how long it takes you to fall asleep
- how many times you wake through the night
- sleep length
- sleep depth
- one word to describe your sleep

Grab your habit tracker and, with the results in mind, write your:

- single thing you are the most proud of overall

- biggest strength regarding your habits and how this impacted your sleep

- biggest challenge regarding your habits and how this impacted your sleep

- how to overcome this challenge this week

Your primary goal for the week ahead, with respect to sleep, how will this impact you:

- mentally
- physically
- at work
- in your relationships

Accountability partner session planner:

- Share your reflections above.

- Go through your habit tracker results.

- After you've read through this week's action plan, do you perceive any roadblocks or limitations?

- If so, how can you overcome this? Map it out.

- If there is one way your AP can support you this week, what is it?

Action plan additions:

- Practise your chronotypes full morning routine at least three days

- Limit two sleep saboteurs: caffeine and alcohol (one coffee a day for Bears and Lions only and two standard drinks across the week, maximum, for all)

- Limit one other sleep saboteur of your choice

WEEK THREE

Okay, you've passed the halfway mark of the twenty-eight-day challenge – how are you feeling? I hope you are following the plan as best as you can, reaching out to your coach for support as you need and, of course, noticing some significant shifts in your sleep.

This week's action plan:

- Complete your weekly progress report above (in the notes from Week Two)

- If you have reached your targets as per your incentive scheme on your habit tracker, reward yourself accordingly

- Have your AP session (as per the outline in Week Two)

- Continue practising your chronotypes full bedtime routine for five days

- Continue taking sleep supplements each day

- Continue to limit two sleep saboteurs: caffeine and alcohol (one coffee a day for Bears and Lions only, and two standard drinks across the week, maximum, for all)

- Continue limiting one other sleep saboteur of your choice (the same as Week Two)

Action plan additions:
- Practise your chronotype's full morning routine at least five days
- Practise at least three days of your chronotype's sleep diet
- Limit one further sleep saboteur of your choice

WEEK FOUR

It's the last week of the twenty-eight-day challenge to make the magic happen – it's your time to shine!

This week's action plan:

- Complete your weekly progress report above (in the notes from Week Two)
- If you have reached your targets as per your incentive scheme on your habit tracker, reward yourself accordingly
- Have your AP session (as per the outline in Week Two)

- Continue practising your chronotype's full bedtime routine for five days

- Continue taking sleep supplements each day

- Continue to limit two sleep saboteurs: caffeine and alcohol (on coffee a day for Bears and Lions only, and two standard drinks across the week, maximum, for all)

- Continue limiting one other sleep saboteur of your choice (the same as Week Two)

- Practise your chronotype's full morning routine at least five days

- Practise at least three days of your chronotype's sleep diet

This week's additions:
- Practise the daytime routine at least three days

- Use your chronotype's aromatherapy through the day

- Book in for your complementary therapy

- Limit one more sleep saboteur of choice

WEEK FIVE – WRAP UP!

First and foremost, I want you to appreciate your efforts. Even if some weeks that meant only a minor improvement in some areas, and perhaps going 'backwards' in others; even if you didn't progress as far as you'd like, the fact is that you're taking action – that is a sign of progress itself. Remember, results aren't created by thinking, they are created by doing.

Be fair on yourself, though – this is your first twenty-eight days and you're trying to rebuild habits that have been established for *years*. Even with the best support, a great system and a deep desire to change, this can be a challenge – to say the least. With this in mind, know that the best results do come when you have these elements in place – so, if you're not seeing a coach or you missed an AP session; or perhaps you forgot to fill in your habit tracker a few nights running, know these small deficits make a big difference.

But rather than play a guessing game, let's assess: how did you *really* go with the twenty-eight-day sleep challenge? What was your highlight, lowlight, your strengths and your weaknesses? What results did you see and what goals did you reach? That's what this week's wrap up is all about.

Answer the points below with reference to the past fortnight.

1. On a scale of 1 to 10, with 10 being the best, rate your:
- sleep quality overall
- ability to fall asleep with ease
- ability to return to sleep, should you wake through the night
- feelings of refreshment upon waking
- energy through the day
- stress and anxiety overall
- stress and anxiety related to sleep
- mental clarity
- memory
- concentration
- motivation at work
- motivation outside of work
- ability to be present with others

2. Specify the following:
- how long it takes you to fall asleep
- how many times you wake through the night

- sleep length

- sleep depth

- one word to describe your sleep

3. Grab your habit tracker and, with last week's results in mind, write your:

- Single thing you are the most proud of

- biggest strength regarding your habits and how this impacted your sleep

- biggest challenge regarding your habits and how this impacted your sleep

- How to overcome this challenge in the future

4. Your primary goal for the week ahead, with respect to sleep (yes, it doesn't stop now!)

5. How will this impact you:

- mentally

- physically

- at work

- in your relationships

Overall

- What was your biggest 'win' from the twenty-eight-day sleep challenge, with regards to your sleep?
- What are the best three changes you've seen in your sleep?
- How has this impacted:
  - Your physical health?
    - And as a result, what are you able to do with greater ease?
  - Your mental health?
    - As a result, what impact do you leave on those around you?
  - Your intimate relationship, family and/or closest friends?
    - How does this change how you 'show up' each day?
    - Are there any specific activities which are more enjoyable for you both now?
    - If so, which ones and how?
  - Your work?
    - What do your colleagues now say about you – as in, what's changed?

- How does this change your interactions with your clients?

- Has your work quality changed and, if so, how?

PART 3

YOUR SLEEP AND YOUR HEALTH

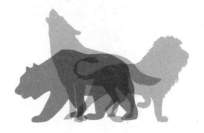

12

SLEEP DISORDERS, DREAMS AND PARASOMNIAS

If you've ever wondered if your sleep is 'normal', this chapter is for you. It covers sleep disorders such as insomnia and sleep apnoea, parasomnias like night terrors and our ever-elusive dreams. Here, I share insight into key symptoms of these conditions. While Wolves are overall the most likely to have these conditions, this doesn't discount the fact that Bears and Lions may suffer as well.

If you are concerned about your sleep and resonate with these hallmark signs, don't delay seeking treatment: as I'm sure you've realised, sleeplessness isn't just a problem at night – it's a problem for your life as a whole. Bears,

Lions and Wolves alike, you deserve to live your best life, filled with your natural, radiant energy. And, as you know, in a sleep-deprived state, this just doesn't happen.

INSOMNIA

The term 'insomnia' is thrown around a lot in pop culture; however, if you are a true insomniac, you appreciate the gravity of the word. Signified by regular and persistent sleep problems for at least a month, one of the most defining symptoms is the lack of restorative sleep. While there are different subtypes of insomnia, as a general rule, those with the condition usually have difficulties falling and staying asleep, wake up unrefreshed and experience daytime fatigue.

So, what are the risk factors? Ongoing exposure to any of the sleep saboteurs mentioned in chapter five, including blue light, devices and stress, will jeopardise your sleep. That said, many of us experience insomnia not through any fault of our own, but from factors beyond our control. As you would have read in chapter three, the ageing process naturally reduces slow-wave sleep (SWS), which contributes to lighter, restless and unrefreshing sleep. Mental health is another major factor.

A 2018 paper by the University of Florida noted that up to 90 per cent of participants with clinical depression also suffered from insomnia, as did 70 per cent of those with generalised anxiety disorder.

Those with an evening preference (Wolves and on-the-cusp Bears) are more likely to suffer from insomnia.

OBSTRUCTIVE SLEEP APNOEA (OSA)

Marked by apnoeas (temporary lapses in breathing during sleep, frequent nighttime wakings, loud snoring and extreme daytime fatigue), mild OSA is a common condition suffered by one in five adults, as noted by researchers at Tulane University School of Medicine in Louisiana, 2009. However, as these symptoms can be difficult to detect, unfortunately up to 85 per cent of cases go undiagnosed.

In terms of predisposing factors, there are a few key considerations. First, simply being a male makes you three times more likely to suffer from OSA, compared to females. If this is coupled with excess weight, the risk grows – those who are obese are seven times more likely to have OSA. A 2012 review indicated that for every 10 per cent increase in weight above the healthy weight range, there was a 32 per cent increase in sleep apnoea severity.

Drinking alcohol, even at a low amount, increases the risk of apnoeas by 29 per cent, as noted in a study published in 2018. The study also found this figure increases to 41 per cent with higher intake of alcohol – so yes, five drinks are worse than one.

NIGHTMARES

I remember the recurring nightmare I had as a little girl. I would be with my mum walking to the shops – when we arrived, she went inside, but a flock of seagulls wouldn't let me in with her and she couldn't hear me. The seagulls would start to attack me and I was left alone, helplessly crying for my mum. While writing this down now makes me laugh a little (I actually love seagulls these days!), I remember as a little girl it was absolutely terrifying.

Occurring in REM sleep and therefore usually after 3am, nightmares are experienced by most of us from time to time and are usually triggered by stress – be it subconscious or conscious. They are particularly common for those who 'bottle up' their emotions, as during sleep your conscious defence mechanisms are down, so nightmares provide a space for your repressed emotions to arise.

NIGHT TERRORS

Although they sound similar, night terrors are very different from nightmares. Firstly, night terrors are extremely rare. Secondly, unlike nightmares, they take place in NREM sleep, typically before 3am. Finally, night terrors are easy to identify – a 'piercing scream', kicking, screaming and sweating are common symptoms. While observers can see the individual is in extreme distress, one of the worst aspects of this parasomnia is that the sufferer is unresponsive to comfort. The best that many parents and caregivers can do is simply wait until the terror resolves itself. Although night terrors are hard to predict and poorly understood, like nightmares, they are thought to be triggered by stress.

SLEEPWALKING

Sleepwalking isn't really an appropriate name – it's much more than just *walking*. Making food, using the bathroom, even reading – sleepwalkers go about their activities as if they were awake. Frighteningly, they truly look like they are awake, with their eyes open. However, they are actually in deep sleep and, as a result, unaware of what they are doing – which can be a danger for themselves and others around them.

Fortunately, only a small subset of the adult population sleepwalks; however, it can be more common in children. Regarding risk factors, stress is at the core: a 2019 paper by Norwegian University of Science and Technology noted 66 per cent of sleepwalkers reported a highly stressful event in the days prior to their episode. Similarly, suffering a psychiatric condition such as anxiety or depression means you are four times more likely to sleepwalk. This is perhaps not surprising, given the interrelationship between these conditions and stress itself. Alcohol is another predisposing factor, as is medication use.

In terms of chronotypes, while there is no evidence so far to pinpoint who is at greatest risk, we can infer that it's most likely to be Wolves, based on the risk factors and their vulnerability to them. Compared to Lions and Bears, they are more likely to suffer from bipolar disorder, depression and feel anxious. Similarly, they are the most likely of any chronotype to use sleep medications and alcohol.

SLEEP TALKING

As with other parasomnias, sleep talking is often linked to stress and is more likely for those with mental health conditions. In addition, like nightmares, sleep talking is experienced by most people at some point in their lives and is nothing to be concerned about.

DREAMS

Dreams are a mystery to us – why do they occur, what do they mean and why can we remember some but not others?

First up, I'm sorry to say that researchers still don't know *why* we dream. Sure, one of the causes may be stress but there isn't a clear correlation. The other thing we all want to know is – what do our dreams *represent*? Again, the unfortunate news is that the research does not tell us much. And finally, do we dream every single night? The answer is believed to be yes. What researchers know for sure is that dreams occur in REM sleep, which is when memory consolidation and emotional processing takes place.

A final note here is reserved for a special type of dream: lucid dreams. They are defined by the ability to control your dream – you have the capacity to act out your wildest dreams (pun intended!): be it time travel, flying on a magic carpet to Bali or trekking through the Amazon. In lucid dreams, it's all possible.

REFLECTION TIME

★ Did you recognise any of the signs of insomnia in yourself? If so, which ones?

★ Are there any other sleep disorders or parasomnias that ring true for you?

★ If yes, how does this affect you, day to day?

★ Do you suspect any of your family or friends suffer from sleep disorders or parasomnias?

★ Do you dream?

★ What is your biggest takeaway from this chapter?

13

HEALTH CONDITIONS LINKED TO POOR SLEEP

One of the reasons I am so passionate about sleep is because of the links between poor sleep and health conditions, particularly mental health. While we all know we feel a little 'off' after insufficient sleep or a restless night, I strongly believe there is a lack of awareness as to the seriousness of sleeplessness. I also recognise that many of us struggle with the challenges of ill health.

With this in mind, I wanted to highlight the interrelationships between sleep and health, and to reassure you that by improving your sleep, you may also be able to improve some other common health conditions.

MOOD DISORDERS
Depression

As many of you may already know, there is strong correlation between depression and poor sleep. A 2008 research paper by the University of Bristol found 97 per cent of participants with depression also reported sleep disturbances. Specifically, 59 per cent of the group woke frequently through the night and 61 per cent woke too early (3 to 4am).

Depression can also worsen when we don't sleep enough – so much so that the degree of mood impairment can reflect the degree of sleep debt. And those with insomnia – the chronically sleep deprived – are six times more likely to later develop depression.

In terms of sleep architecture, those with depression spend more time in REM sleep, less time in slow-wave sleep and have a circadian phase delay – typically, they sleep and wake later than normal. As you would remember, this sleeping pattern is characteristic of Wolves. In fact, a 2013 paper in *Chronobiology International* found Wolves are up to four times more likely to be depressed than Lions, and almost twice as likely to be depressed than Bears.

Anxiety/anxiety disorders

Though it's been mentioned extensively, it's important to underline the connection between anxiety and sleeplessness. As I mentioned in chapter one, research by the University of Chicago found that just one night of inadequate sleep can see the stress hormone cortisol increase by 37 per cent. So, it's no wonder that after a night of insufficient sleep, you might be feeling anxious, alert and 'wired' the next day – and this can feed into the following night too.

Long term, sleeplessness and anxiety continue to propel each other. A 2013 paper in the journal *Sleep* noted that insomniacs are seventeen times more likely to have an anxiety disorder and that up to 70 per cent of those with generalised anxiety disorder (GAD) also have symptoms of insomnia.

With respect to chronotypes, as mentioned previously, Wolves are at greatest risk. It's worth noting, however, that Lions can also be prone to anxiety and that just because Bears are the least likely to suffer, doesn't mean they don't. After all, anxiety is experienced by most people from time to time.

Bipolar disorder

Bipolar is a condition where the sufferer experiences periods of depression and periods of mania, with periods of stable mood in between. With regards to sleep, there is a strong correlation between bipolar and sleep issues – a 2016 Harvard Medical School review found that 99 per cent of participants with bipolar struggled to fall or stay asleep in a manic state, whereas during a depressive phase, 78 per cent overslept. Furthermore, between phases, 70 per cent experienced sleep disturbances. The evidence also indicated that insufficient sleep exacerbated bipolar symptoms.

Post-traumatic stress disorder (PTSD)

Sleep and stress are inextricably intertwined, so it comes as no surprise that researchers have found links between sleep and PTSD. In fact, findings published in the medical journal *CNS Drugs* noted that 91 per cent of those with PTSD have difficulty falling and staying asleep, and that the severity of the trauma can often reflect the severity of the sleeping problem.

Unfortunately, even when they do sleep, those with PTSD face an uphill battle – they typically spend a higher portion of their sleep time in Stage 1 NREM (light sleep), have less slow-wave sleep, too much REM sleep and experience parasomnias such as nightmares and night terrors.

Panic attacks

I've experienced panic attacks a few times and they are absolutely horrible. Think racing heart, sweating and a feeling that the world is about to implode. While mine have occurred during the day, I can only imagine how traumatic this is when it happens at night.

A 2003 paper in the journal *Dialogues in Clinical Neuroscience* found 68 per cent of participants who suffered from panic attacks had difficulty falling asleep and 77 per cent had disturbed, restless sleep. In addition, 67 per cent of participants who suffered from panic attacks also had insomnia.

As panic attacks are a subset of anxiety disorders, it's likely that Wolves will more commonly experience them, compared to Bears and Lions.

SUBSTANCE ABUSE

Alcohol

As highlighted in chapter five, alcohol is, without a doubt, problematic for sleep – especially if it turns into abuse.

Research by University Hospitals in Ohio in 2009 found that 97 per cent of those who are alcohol dependent also report high levels of sleep disturbance. As you may remember from chapter five, even mild consumption of alcohol suppresses REM sleep and compromises sleep quality – and the more alcohol in your system, the worse the suppression.

On the other hand, a 2015 paper by Idaho State University found that those who have trouble sleeping are up to 65 per cent more likely to binge drink. So, we can see that these two conditions – sleeplessness and alcoholism – perpetuate each other.

Regarding chronotypes, research in *Chronobiology International* in 2012 indicates that Wolves are more likely to use and abuse alcohol than Bears or Lions.

EATING DISORDERS

Anorexia nervosa and bulimia nervosa

Having only recently overcome a decade-plus battle with anorexia, I know from personal experience that eating disorders affect *everything*, including sleep. A 2010 study by Yonsei University in Korea found 50 per cent of those with eating disorders – specifically anorexia and bulimia – experience sleep disturbances, typically having lighter, less restorative sleep and sleeping less. The study also found that those with anorexia and bulimia often have an abnormal circadian cycle – 25 per cent have an extreme early phase (sleeping before 9pm and waking by 5am), and another 20 per cent have an extreme late phase (sleeping after 1am and waking after 9am).

There are a few reasons for this. Firstly, anorexics are often nutrient deprived and, as you may recall, this is a significant sleep saboteur. Similarly, those with eating disorders, particularly bulimia, often have gut problems, which may compromise their nutritional absorption and their sleep in the process. Finally, those suffering from eating disorders often have a mood disorder as well, which further increases their risk of poor sleep.

Excess weight: obesity and overweight

There is a link between your weight and the quality of your sleep. A 2019 study published in *Nature and Science of Sleep* found that those with obesity are 67 per cent more likely to experience poor sleep quality and twice as likely to sleep less than six hours a night, compared to those who are a healthy weight. However, similar results have been observed in those who are overweight too.

On the other hand, insufficient sleep has been shown to encourage weight gain. As mentioned in chapter one, a 2004 study by the University of Chicago found that after just two nights of inadequate sleep, the hunger hormone ghrelin increased by 28 per cent, the satiety hormone leptin decreased by 18 per cent and cravings for sugary carbohydrates increased by up to 45 per cent.

PHYSICAL CONDITIONS

Gut disorders: GERD/IBS

As you may recall from chapter eight, a healthy microbiome can support sleep. And, as you can imagine, those with compromised gut integrity – be it from gastroesophageal reflux disease (GERD) or irritable bowel disease (IBS) – are more likely to experience subpar sleep. In fact, research by Ewha Womans University in Korea in 2010 found that 49 per cent of those with GERD symptoms such as heartburn struggled to fall asleep and 58 per cent found it difficult to stay asleep. Similarly, 57 per cent of those with IBS also reported disrupted sleep, with the evidence indicating that the worse their symptoms, the worse their sleep quality.

However, often, inadequate sleep can precede these

conditions too – a 2015 paper published by George Washington University highlighted that insomniacs are three times more likely to suffer from GERD.

Yet again, the conditions seem to feed each other. This makes sense – lack of sleep reduces healthy gut bacteria, compromising our ability to produce the happiness hormone serotonin, and therefore melatonin. It also compromises our ability to absorb key micronutrients we need for sleep, such as Omega-3s.

With insufficient sleep commonplace for Wolves, they are at particular risk for these illnesses and should be extra careful to protect their gut health, and sleep health, collectively.

Type 2 diabetes

For Wolves, I'm sorry to say, there's more unfortunate news: a 2019 paper by Northumbria University reported you are 2.5 times more likely than other chronotypes to have Type 2 diabetes. That said, Bears and Lions are also at risk, should they not be getting enough sleep – a 2015 study led by Chang Gung University in Taiwan found that those sleeping less than five hours per night were five times more likely to develop Type 2 diabetes than those sleeping seven to nine hours. Yes, *five times*.

Irrespective of chronotype, insufficient sleep and diabetes are closely intertwined. Sleep deprivation leads to insulin resistance, which encourages a higher sugar intake and likely weight gain – all factors which increase the risk of Type 2 diabetes.

Cardiovascular disease

As one of the leading killers globally, we all need to do what we can to reduce our risk of cardiovascular disease. A 2006 paper published by the Institute of Medicine in Washington noted that sleeping less than five hours per night increases your likelihood of a heart attack by a staggering 45 per cent. Furthermore, the evidence also indicates the more severe your sleep loss, the greater your risk.

In terms of chronotypes, a research paper by North-western University in Chicago noted the more evening-oriented you are, the greater the risk for cardiovascular disease – so, Wolves, take note. But Bears and Lions are not exempt from the risk, either. A 2014 study by the University of Colorado showed that disruptions in sleeping patterns can increase the risk of heart attacks – and this applies to any chronotype.

Chronic pain

As many of us know, chronic pain conditions such as arthritis and fibromyalgia can compromise sleep. Not only does chronic pain leave you tossing and turning all night, it also increases the need for sleep saboteur medications such as codeine, morphine and aspirin. In addition, as noted in a 2017 paper published by Jilin University in China, 85 per cent of those with chronic pain suffer depression, which then indirectly increases the risk of problematic sleep.

In terms of chronotypes, the more evening-oriented you are, the more likely you are to experience inflammation, as well as conditions such as fibromyalgia, osteoarthritis and rheumatoid arthritis. That said, many of these conditions are genetic, so this may be relevant to many Lions and Bears as well.

Infertility

Falling pregnant and having a baby is *meant* to be one of the most joyful times in your life . . . unless it doesn't happen naturally. Though I haven't been through this myself, after hearing stories of heartbreak from friends and family, I deeply empathise with those who struggle with fertility – I can only imagine how saddening it must be. With this in mind, I'm inspired to share what I know about sleep with a view to helping you and your partner.

Statistically, adequate sleep is important – for both sexes. For women, a 2002 study published in the journal *Fertility and Sterility* highlighted that women sleeping eight or more hours had 20 per cent more follicle stimulating hormone (FSH; a hormone which helps control the menstrual cycle and the production of eggs by the ovaries), compared to women sleeping less than eight hours. For men, a 2017 study by Baylor College of Medicine in Texas found that males sleeping insufficiently – that is, sleeping only five hours per night over the course of a week – produced 10 to 15 per cent less testosterone, compared to when they attained more sleep.

Alzheimer's disease (AD)

After witnessing my dear nonna struggle with Alzheimer's disease, I know how painful it is for the sufferer and for those around them. Unfortunately, if you have sleeping issues, your risk of developing the condition increases by 51 per cent, as noted in a 2020 report by the University of Valencia in Spain.

As mentioned a few times before, a primary factor here is beta-amyloid (Aβ), a neurotoxin that contributes to impaired memory, and has been linked to a lack of sleep. A 2018 paper by National Institutes of Health, USA, noted that just *one* night of inadequate sleep increases Aβ levels by 5 per cent. When a lack of sleep becomes chronic, Aβ can continue to build up in the brain and form plaques, which causes even greater memory loss and is a hallmark of Alzheimer's.

With respect to chronotypes, at the time of writing, there is no significant correlation between this illness and a specific circadian preference.

REFLECTION TIME

★ Do you suffer from any of these health conditions? If so, which ones?

★ Do you notice that the symptoms of your condition become worse if you've had a bad night's sleep, or a few bad nights?

★ Did any of the research findings surprise you?

★ What is your biggest takeaway from this chapter?

CLOSING NOTES

I wanted to finish the book by thanking you for coming this far and trusting me on this journey to improve your sleep and, hopefully, your life. Whether you are going to do everything, or just one thing, all I ask is that you do *something*.

If there is one thing I know, it's that change comes from *action*, not intention. I also know that deep down, that's why we are here: to change. To grow, to evolve, to become our best selves. And I truly believe that by using these strategies, taking my advice and getting the support you need, that *will* happen.

You'll start to sleep more, live more, be more.

You'll start to become that version of yourself that you truly want to be: one with energy, enthusiasm and a radiant glow. I know that that person is within you, and also know that when you are getting the sleep you need, you will see that, too.

Lastly, I want you to see this as the start of our time together, not the end. Feel free to connect with me via email (enquiries@oliviaarezzolo.com.au) or Instagram (@oliviaarezzolo). If there's one thing that I truly want, it is to connect with you – and share the highs and lows of your journey ahead.

Remember, the time is now and the only person who can change your life is you. You have all the tools you need – your personalised chronotype strategy, my support and the opportunity to start using these tools tonight – to get the sleep you deserve.

Sleep well, my friends – Bears, Lions and Wolves alike.

Love from Olivia, your very own sleep coach.

ACKNOWLEDGEMENTS

To my mum, whose ongoing love, support and encouragement has allowed me to become the Lion I am today.

To my fellow Lion dad, who enjoys the crack of dawn as much as I do – Sunday mornings will always have a special place in my heart, as will memories of markets and garage sales with you.

To my puppy Jackie, who reminds me of the true joys in life: a walk, a park, a big stick. I hope I can be as grateful for these simple pleasures as you are.

To my brother, Damon, and his partner, Mel, whose new baby will mean that they, of all my family, may need this book the most.

To my Lion grandma and Bear grandad, whose trials and tribulations in life inspire me in my own adventures – this book included.

To my nonna, who is now in heaven making pasta. And to my nonno, who's currently probably on the farm picking beans, thank you for letting me know that no matter when, I can always pop in and say hello.

To my best friends Lara and Vik – catch ups with you both got me through the writing of this book

To my coaches, Tom and Jeff, who helped me transform myself, so I can be here to transform others.

To my favourite sleep clients, who have opened their hearts and minds and let me change their lives, inspiring me to do more of my coaching in the process. You know who you are.

And lastly, to you. For being here, with me, sharing time, sharing knowledge, sharing this moment. For investing in becoming your best *you*, and allowing me to take you there.

REFERENCES

For a full list of the references used in this book, please refer to my website: oliviaarezzolo.com.au

GLOSSARY

beta-amyloid (Aβ)   a small part of a larger protein called 'amyloid precursor protein' (APP). Beta-amyloid can accumulate into microscopic plaques that are considered a hallmark of a brain affected by Alzheimer's

cortisol   a hormone produced in the body by the adrenal glands; it is mainly released at times of stress

dopamine   a neurotransmitter produced in the brain and strongly associated with pleasure and reward

GABA   gamma-aminobutyric acid; a neurotransmitter that sends chemical messages through the

	brain and nervous system. It plays an important role in the body's response to stress
ghrelin	an important digestive hormone that controls appetite
HGH	human growth hormone; this hormone is produced by the pituitary gland and governs height, bone length and muscle growth
leptin	a hormone produced by the body's fat cells that is crucial to appetite and weight control; often referred to as the 'satiety hormone'
melatonin	a hormone produced in the brain that regulates the sleep-and-wake cycle; it can also be taken as a supplement
REM	short for 'rapid eye movement', also called paradoxical sleep. The brain is highly active during REM sleep, with alpha, beta and gamma brainwaves in action – the latter

being most active. On average, we spend 25 per cent of our sleep time here, primarily in the last third of the evening

sleep inertia	the feeling of grogginess, disorientation, drowsiness and cognitive impairment that may occur immediately after waking
sleep latency	the length of time it takes to make the transition from full wakefulness to sleep
stage 1 NREM	the sleep stage that occurs right after you fall asleep and is very short (usually less than ten minutes); it involves light sleep from which you can be awakened easily
stage 2 NREM	during this stage, awakenings do not occur as easily as stage 1, your body temperature drops and your breathing and heart rate become more regular; the brain also begins to produce bursts of brain wave activity which are known as sleep

	spindles – these are thought to be a feature of memory consolidation
stage 3+4 NREM	also known as slow-wave sleep (SWS); deep, slow brain waves known as delta waves begin to emerge in this stage. It usually occurs in the first two-thirds of the night (typically before 3am) and is critical for both mental and physical recovery
zeitgeber	an environmental agent or event (such as the occurrence of light or dark) that influences your circadian rhythm

INDEX